MW01145883

CANCER

YOUR ROAD
BACK TO HEALTH

Norm Hacker

Copyright © 2014 World Healers LLC

All rights reserved.

No part of this publication may be reproduced in any form or by any electronic or mechanical means, including information storage and retrieval systems, or transmitted, in any form, or by any means (electronic, mechanical, photocopying, recording or otherwise) without prior permission in writing from the author. The only exception is by a reviewer, who may quote short excerpts in a review.

Printed in the United States of America

First Printing: July 2014

ISBN: 978-0-9905334-0-5

IMPORTANT: PLEASE READ

The texts contained herein were compiled over a four year period, as part of the documentary "Heal Your Self". We were committed to retaining as much of the interview flow as possible, which resulted in some of the colloquial phrases that were used.

Within the candid interview setting, there may be certain discussions with regard to medical situations that SHOULD NOT be taken as medical advice. At best, they may be considered as opinions. This information is NOT intended to replace the services of a physician, nor does it constitute a doctor-patient relationship. Information is provided for enlightenment purposes only and is not a substitute for professional medical advice. Readers should not use the information herein for diagnosing or treating a medical or health condition.

You should consult a health care professional in all matters relating to your health, particularly in respect to any symptoms that may require diagnosis or medical attention. Any action on your part in response to the information provided is solely at you, the reader's, discretion.

World Healers LLC, the producers of "Heal Your Self" and of this publication, make no representations or warranties with respect to any information offered or provided on or through these pages or associated links, regarding treatment, action, or application of medication. Certain opinions expressed within these pages may differ from those of World Healers LLC and its associates.

Contents

John Gray, Ph.D.

Health Researcher
Author

Everybody knows me as the author of <u>Men Are From Mars, Woman Are From Venus</u>. What they're not always aware of is that I have a background as a health researcher, and even before I got in the field of <u>Men Are From Mars, Woman Are From Venus</u>, I was a health researcher. Ever since I was a young child, I was doing yoga. I used to teach yoga in my 20s, advocating a vegetarian diet, fasting and cleansing back then.

Then as I moved into relationships, I shifted from just coaching people about their health to coaching them about their relationships, and of course, I wrote a very famous book that I'm very well known for. But I've continued focusing on my understanding of how to create health; my specialty being gender-related health. Because very few people really have the gender insight that I have, I created a variety of different programs to assist men and women in promoting optimal brain chemistry.

Under stress, men have a different reaction than women. If we can understand how we each react differently to stress, then we can take certain steps in our diet, exercise routine, and lifestyle choices to make sure we have optimal brain chemistry. This will lower stress levels in our bodies, which promotes optimal health.

Without a doubt, the rise of cancer in our society, as well as heart disease, diabetes, and autoimmune diseases is directly linked to the increasing levels of stress in our lives and our inability to cope effectively with that stress. Now, often to the layman - when you talk about stress - he starts thinking about rising real estate prices, traffic jams, in-laws, neighbors, those variety of stressors.

But, as a researcher, that's not what we mean regarding how stress causes sickness. What we mean is that when you have stressors - and we all have them in our lives, nobody can escape it today - how does our body react to that? You can, for example, measure that reaction in your adrenal glands by the excretion of adrenalin.

Everybody knows that when you're getting a speeding ticket, your adrenalin level goes up. But, what you don't realize at those times is that all of your basic immune system shuts down for a temporary amount of time. Also, cortisol levels rise, and you can measure cortisol levels in the blood. As people get older in our society, typically their cortisol levels get higher and higher and higher, which means that it's normal for your cortisol level to go way up. Think of it like this: If you get a speeding ticket, your cortisol levels go high. However, these levels of cortisol should come back down. Ours don't come back down completely, however. They slowly, gradually rise up and up, with increasing levels of stress in our bodies, as measured by cortisol.

Our immune systems are compromised, our digestion is compromised, and our ability to remove toxins is compromised, further increasing stress in our lives because of an ineffective way to cope with that stress. We also have these stressors of pollution, toxins in the environment, the amount of chlorine and fluoride, which are both in the water, and pesticides, which are in our food. The literally thousands and thousands of chemicals that are in the air today, and in the last hundred years, didn't exist before.

When these chemicals come into our bodies, that becomes a stressor, and our bodies have a reaction to that as well. And, all of these stress reactions tend to produce acid in the body. Excessive acid is your body's defense mechanism to toxic influences. When you have excessive acid that prevents oxygen from getting to cells - when oxygen is restricted in its ability to get to our cells - cancer will grow.

So we have different stressors, such as emotional stressors which are in our own personal lives - chronic fear, chronic anger, grief, despair, hopelessness, depression, rage - all those types of things are emotional stressors inside of us. This, of course, is going to inhibit the immune system from fighting off cancer and the growth of cancer in the body. However, you also have environmental stressors, whereby the toxins and pollutants are coming into our bodies and we don't have a way of helping our bodies to remove them. This will also weaken and compromise our immune systems.

Now, what's important for people to know is that anybody over forty - if you did an autopsy on this person - you'll find cancer in his or her body. That doesn't mean this person is going to die of cancer; it does mean that cancer is there and that the immune system is keeping it in check. It's when the cancer becomes more powerful than the immune system, that's when cancer has out-of-control growth. That's when it's lethal. Otherwise, it's not a problem; our body is always handling problems. It's like this: life has got problems, our immune system is dealing with those problems, and one of them is the growth of cancer. Also, cancer particularly grows when cells don't get enough oxygen. When cells don't get enough oxygen, then the anaerobic bacteria - that means bacteria that grow in a non-oxygen environment - overpopulate. When they overpopulate at a given period of time, this bacterium begins damaging cells and then cancer will begin to grow. It can grow very quickly sometimes. Conversely, sometimes it's very slow growing.

If you have a strong immune system, your immune system produces killer cells that will come into compromised cells to literally spray oxygen on the anaerobic bacteria and reduce their growth. Each cell can then come back to normal functioning. So one of the things we want to make sure of, in order to avoid cancer in our lives, is to make sure we are properly oxygenating ourselves. We need to make sure our lifestyle choices ensure getting enough oxygen to the cells by not putting up roadblocks to oxygen. Those roadblocks would be creating stress reactions during the day, staying very stressed, or having pollutants come into our bodies. Realistically, they're some pollutants we can't escape; so, what we have to do is to find practical methods to allow the body, help the body, to remove those pollutants.

When someone gets a diagnosis that they have a fast growing cancer, then they have to take fast action. One of the things that you can do is to identify in the last year if any type of extremely stressful event occurred, go see a therapist, and start processing that stressful event. This is very common that people experience heart disease or cancer - particularly those two - within a year there was some big upset. It could be the loss of child, it could be an accident, it could be a loss of money, a bump to your pride, whatever it could be, a break up in a relationship, a divorce.

Any of these types of stresses, emotional stresses, compromise our immune systems. Imagine if something really devastating happened in your life to someone you love or to yourself. Either way, it's happening to you because it's affecting someone you love. This can increase your cortisol levels and the cortisol levels will restrict your body's ability to hold cancer down.

So, suddenly cancer gets a foothold and starts taking off, but at any time we can say, "Okay, let me begin helping my body cope with this." The psychological reduction of stress in our lives can have a huge impact.

When I first start talking about toxins, people really don't understand that it's kind of abstract. I want to give a clear story that people can relate to. I was once with one of my limousine drivers - he was in his 70s - and while we were talking, he was smoking. I was giving him a little talk saying smoking can cause cancer and maybe it's not a good idea for him to smoke. He said, "I've heard the whole story; I've been hearing it for years. I actually gave up smoking." I said, "Well, what happened?" He said, "Well, my grandchildren said, 'Please Grandpa, don't smoke. We want you to live a long healthy life.'" So, for his grandchildren, he gave up smoking. Then in two weeks, he grew a huge tumor in his throat. "This big," he said to me. I said, "Wow, that's amazing," and I said, "What did you do then?" He said, "Well, if I'm going to die of cancer, I might as well die smoking." So, he started smoking again and in two weeks his tumor went away.

Now that's an amazing story. I'm just giving one. I have many examples like that. The concept here is he was smoking cigarettes, which besides tobacco smoke, cigarettes have two hundred and fifty chemicals in them that are toxic to the body. So, you're breathing in all these chemicals, and as they come in, your body's saying, "Okay. To prevent myself from dying, I need to store those chemicals somewhere - those toxins somewhere."

They get stored in tissues, whereby they get pushed away from the organs so the organs aren't compromised by having all these chemicals and toxins. So, they get pushed into our tissues; they get pushed into fat cells; they get hidden around the body. That's called storing and building up toxins, which is what happens to people as they get older. So, he's giving up smoking, and as soon as he stops putting in two hundred and fifty chemicals every day, what does his body want to do? It's now going to start releasing two hundred and fifty chemicals. They're going to start coming out. This happens because the body is already designed to get rid of chemicals.

All we have to do is stop putting them in and the body will start getting rid of them. So immediately his system started dumping chemicals into the blood system, toxins into the blood system. He was becoming toxic by giving up putting toxins in his body.

So I said to him, "If you give up smoking, your body is going to start detoxifying. Did you drink lots of water?" He said, "Yes." And I said, "Tell me what kind of water." He said, "Well I drank coffee." I laughed, I said to him, "Coffee has water in it, but coffee has a dehydrating effect. So anything that dehydrates your cells does not promote removing toxins from the cells." In the infinite intelligence of the body - the body is very smart - it said, "I have to protect myself from these toxins, so I'm going to grow a tumor." And that's what the tumors do.

Tumors collect toxins in them, protecting the organs

from the body's chemicals. If you ever pull a tumor out of someone, you'll find that it's filled with toxic chemicals. It's like a miniature liver. When your liver is over-burdened, and your liver can't pull all of the toxins out because it's already too toxic, then your body will begin growing tumors to absorb those toxins. All this man had to do was to start smoking again, which started getting chemicals to his body. His body stopped releasing chemicals and the tumor went away.

I'm not recommending smoking to people to take away tumors. What I'm pointing out is that there's a cause and effect in the relationship between cigarettes and tumors. When you're adding chemicals and toxins into your body, your body is storing them. So when you start thinking about removing these toxins, you need to do it very wisely. There are a variety of different cleansing approaches to do that. We have to be very wise in that process. Now, if we don't cleanse our bodies, there does come a point where, even if we continue absorbing toxins, our bodies are going to become too toxic and cancer will grow. Tumors will develop as a way to isolate those toxins, which can't be stored anymore.

Think about the house having several closets in it to store your junk. That's what the tissues and the fat cells of the body are for. So, the body will just store toxins away. But, at a certain point, it can't store anymore. Your house becomes a mess. That's when you start getting tumors, and then as those toxins get isolated in tumors, cancer has a chance to grow if you don't find some way of cleansing the body.

I've seen many programs which are very alkaline promoting, and that helps to rebalance the body from an acid state to a more alkaline state. Just like if you have a hot tub, you have to balance certain chemicals. You can add something to make the acid go up, or you can add something to make the acid go down, so the water becomes more base or alkaline.

The body has to be more alkaline, or has to have the right balance of alkaline and acid. The alkalinity is what delivers oxygen to the cells. When you don't have enough alkalinity, then you can't get enough oxygen to your cells. And without enough oxygen to your cells, cancer has a chance to grow. So there are programs where you can follow certain alkaline producing diets, which are very, very helpful.

For example a meat free diet will promote alkalinity. I don't say someone has to go on this kind of diet; it's just one of the routes you can go on. But, I often see people giving up meat thinking, "Okay, I'm giving up a big acid producer," because meat does produce some acid ash in the body. It's not necessarily that significant, but it is significant to some degree. But people will go to great lengths to go on a meat free diet, for example, and put all kinds of alkaline producing foods in their diet, which is good. Then they go out and have a candy bar on their day off. That candy bar will negate the effects of everything.

Your major acid producer is refined sugars. Anything which has corn syrup in it, fructose in it - this is processed fructose not just regular fruit - any of these processed sugars, concentrated sugars, has a huge acid effect in the body compared to the little effect that meat products have in the food we eat. People have been eating meat for thousands of years and cancer wasn't around, so I don't see eating meat as a cause of cancer. What I see as the major cause of cancer today is the amount of processed foods that people are eating. Stress on one hand, and processed foods on the other, lead to cancer. And, of course, it's the stress that makes us want to eat processed foods. Once we eat processed foods, it actually raises our stress levels.

So for me, somebody might say I have a very stressful life, lots of stressors, but I'm not stressed about it because I don't eat processed foods. If I eat a processed food that begins to disturb the acid/alkaline balance in my body, it causes insulin levels to spike. It causes sugar levels to increase in my body, which then prevent my body from burning fat for energy. Then suddenly, I run out of energy faster. I'm craving more sugar and that's the loop people get into.

Sugar products provide fast, easy energy; they make your brain feel really good. They make you feel optimistic; they make you feel happy. But, just like kindling wood in a fireplace, you put it in and it burns fast. Because it burns easy, it burns out real fast. Then, you need more and more and more. The problem with that is the by-product of eating refined sugar products is lactic acid. You produce way too much lactic acid and your body can't get rid of it. Your body can't process it, and then your body is filled with more acid and less alkalinity.

Clearly, if you wanted to name one of the major causes of cancer - and I see this sometimes in the papers stating causes of cancer - this was discovered a long time ago. This is so clear: it's the rise of sugar consumption in this country. Sugar is in every packaged food, because packagers know that if they put corn syrup, fructose sugar - high levels of sugar in everything, including ketchup and pickles - it makes food addictive. Everything's got sugar in it if it's a packaged food. Suppliers all have it in there because of the addiction factor, and if you don't have that in your food, nobody's going to buy your product. If consumers eat your product, they're going to go, "That was really good, and when I have this, I want more."

So sugar is known by manufacturers to create a greater draw in the audience. I don't think they're planning to go and cause cancer for everybody, but it's the number one contributor to cancer in our bodies. When we eat more than a couple of teaspoons of sugar at a time, this is the problem. Two teaspoons equal about eight grams, but almost everything we buy has more than eight grams in it. Everything always has twenty or thirty grams of sugar. What that will do is raise our blood sugar to dangerously high levels, so our body compensates.

It goes into an emergency mode of burning up all that sugar, so it stops burning fat. It burns sugar for energy, and the by-product for all that sugar burning to create energy is lactic acid. That then becomes the problem. How does your body get rid of that acid?

Some people's bodies, what they do to compensate, is they will store lactic acid in fat cells. Other people's bodies pull the calcium out of the bones in order to neutralize the acids. Then, you have osteoporosis. And different body types will do different things; however, in all those situations you're creating an environment where your body is less alkaline and your potential for getting cancer dramatically goes up.

And this is not just sugar products causing issues, let me remind you. It's also refined carbohydrates. Anything that you buy in the store - breads, rolls, cakes, even whole wheat bread - just look at. It's processed bread. Unless it's like really clumpy, the way bread used to be a long time ago - most people don't even remember that - you will have to chew it for a while before it breaks down. This bread is processed, it's refined. And, if it's refined bread, it instantly turns right into glucose into your blood stream.

Whenever your glucose levels are too quick, too high, then your muscles begin burning the sugar for energy and you get lactic acid. Better to have a little bit of sugar in your system, and then your body will burn fat for energy. That's the healthy state.

There are a whole different variety of types of sweeteners, and they're not all bad. The way you understand sweeteners, making sure you don't have a negative effect from them, is watching how much you have of them. Let's just look at it. There's evaporated cane sugar, probably one of your best sugars. The brain needs sugar for energy, by the way. We need some glucose. So, you're getting evaporated cane sweetener, which is cane sugar and what's left in it - the minerals. So that's a plus - you're getting good minerals. Basically, with that kind of a sweetener, you're getting the minerals your body needs to utilize that sugar. As long as you have it in a moderate amount, it's going to have no negative effect. If you had thirty grams of that kind of sugar, which is a good sugar, thirty grams would be way too much. More than a few teaspoons on an empty stomach are too much.

There's a certain range when your blood sugar is at a moderate level. At this point, the brain uses all that sugar and the muscles burn fat for energy. As soon as sugar goes to dangerously high levels, which means more than a couple of teaspoons in your blood system, it's floating around. Then, your body's sugar levels are too high; so let's lower them. And the way your body lowers those sugar levels is by getting the muscles to now burn sugar for energy. When the muscles burn sugar, the by-product is lactic acid. And, that's where the danger is.

So keep in mind that anything which is producing too much lactic acid is making your body too acidic. A small amount of cane sugar is great. A small amount of honey is great. A small amount of brown sugar is okay as well. Now you've got two types of brown sugar. You've got real brown sugar, which is made from sugar cane containing molasses - where they haven't taken refined white sugar and simply added molasses to it. A lot of the brown sugar today is refined white sugar that has had molasses put on it. Molasses is a very fine sweetener, which I use a lot. Molasses is left when they make refined sugar from sugar beets or sugar cane. The processing pulls out all of the minerals and some of the sugar comes out of it as well, and that's what molasses is. So, that's your healthy sweetener. Your healthiest choice is molasses. Evaporated cane sugar is also in the "healthiest" category.

Then, you get into refined sugars. Even when you have refined sugar at a moderate amount, it's still unhealthy for the body. That's because you're putting sugar into the body, and when the brain uses that sugar, it requires minerals in your body to metabolize it. If you ingest refined sugar, the brain has to use its storehouse of minerals to burn it, instead of the minerals that were naturally part of the sugar. So, that's additional insight when it comes to sugar.

So, your unhealthy sugars, the sugars to avoid, are those dangerous sugars all made from corn syrup, corn sugars, fructose, and high-fructose. These are highly refined, processed, and concentrated sugars. They go right into the system and they cause your blood sugar levels to go really high, which then causes the burning of sugar and the creation of lactic acid and so forth. There are many other negative side effects of sugar, but from the point of view of acid, those are some of the basic ideas.

When someone is diagnosed with cancer, immediately this individual wants to ask: "How have I contributed to creating this disease?" And we have, we always have. There are three major areas to look at. There's the emotional component; there's the nutritional component - what are we putting into our bodies? How are we exposing ourselves to different toxins and literally eating and drinking them? A third component is simply the environmental effects. For example, one of the causes I support is to help children who were born with cancer. How does a child get born with cancer when his parents don't have cancer? They say we don't know, except that all these children happen to grow up on farms where they use pesticides. To me, it's as clear as day - it's the toxic effect of pesticides. This is why there's a movement to encourage a more organic lifestyle, which means not using pesticides because they cause cancer, period. Eating foods grown and treated with pesticides contributes to cancer, so that's one aspect to consider.

But, more insidious and more all permeating is the water we drink. The water we bathe in is also a major contributor to cancer. What we have to understand, for example, is that where I live here in the San Francisco Bay Area, Marin County, we're well known as the most affluent county in the world. We were also known in the 70s as the hot tub capital of the world. Now, we're known as the breast cancer capital of the world. I see a clear link between the two.

Affluence links breast cancer and hot tubs. The nature of the environment and the climate here is such that we have swimming pools, but we don't use them that often. It's a bit too cold for the swimming pool. But, we have leisure time, due to an affluent lifestyle, to spend time in our hot tubs. The water is very relaxing and it's a very healthy thing to spend time in a hot tub, except that the water we use is toxic.

In order to keep that water clean, smelling nice and looking nice, people have used the most popular method, which is chlorinating the water. When you put chlorine in water, this chlorine is a toxic substance to the body. When chlorine goes in and then you put jets on, you're creating chlorine gas - which happens to be very relaxing and sedating - but it's toxic to the body. It turns out that Marin County has the highest rate of breast cancer and the highest number of hot tubs.

This is happening in everybody's home when they take a shower. When you take a shower and your water is chlorinated, that chlorine in the water going through the jet stream of the shower spray will turn to gas. It's the chlorine gas that permeates through your whole body. The problem with chlorine, fluoride, and bromine in drinking water is that those are three basic elements that the body cannot distinguish individually. These three elements, along with iodine, are indistinguishable in order for the body to purify itself and keep down the anaerobic bacterial growth. We mentioned that anaerobic bacteria over-populate and cancer grows.

One of the ways the body keeps the anaerobic bacteria from over-populating is with iodine. Every fourteen minutes, all of the blood in your body goes through the thyroid gland. The thyroid gland collects iodine from the food we eat, and the thyroid then uses that iodine to kill bad bacteria. Just like if you had a cut, you put iodine on it to keep the bad bacteria from over-populating and causing a problem.

When you're exposed to chlorine on a regular basis, chlorine goes into the body. This chlorine will go to the iodine receptor sites and prevent the receptor sites from absorbing iodine. So what happens? They've done tests on breast cancer, proving women who have breast cancer have extremely low levels of iodine in their breasts. There are three major places that our bodies store iodine. One place is in the thyroid gland, another one is in the breasts, and a third place is in the uterus for women and the prostate for men.

What I would encourage people to do is to immediately get filters on their showers, which are very inexpensive and easily obtainable. Filters will neutralize the effects of the chlorine in the shower and bathtubs as well. Stores sell little balls you can run through your bathtub that will neutralize the effects of chlorine. So, you can easily take Jacuzzi baths and get the beneficial effect, rather than the cancer causing effect.

When I'm talking about water, I always want to mention the water we drink. People who drink tap water are exposing themselves to a variety of toxins, as well as the chlorine and the fluoride - which both have a toxic effect on the body and will gradually promote cancer. On one hand, we're looking at all the packaged foods and the sugar and refined carbohydrates that will immediately throw the body into an acid state rather than an alkaline state. We also have to look at the high consumption of coffee, which will put the body into an acid state rather than an oxygen state. We have to look at tap water, which is filled with all kinds of toxins, including chlorine and fluoride, that inhibit the use of iodine in the body to fight cancer. The water we ingest is highly, highly important. Drinking purified water is essentially very, very important.

With over thirty years' experience as a health researcher myself, I've seen a variety of different pathways for people who have healed their cancer - have gone into remission with their cancer. Personally, for myself, I've led various types of groups through this process. One group I led, I advertised in the paper: "Spend time with Dr. John Gray, author of <u>Men Are From Mars, Women Are From Venus</u>. Learn his health secrets." I invited only people who were in Stage 4 cancer. Basically, they had to be given up by their doctors to die. They were done with the chemotherapy and done with the radiation, as it didn't work. Then I took them in my course for free. This was a six-week program.

Within the first week, five people died. They couldn't do any of the things I recommended; they were on morphine at that point. There was nothing I could do for them or help them do for themselves. Within the three-month program, within probably six weeks to eight weeks, we had fifteen people go into complete remission. Then, of the remaining people, nobody got worse and everybody got better.

To this day, where I live, people walk up to me in the grocery store and say, "Hi remember me?" I say, "No." They say, "It's because I have hair now." Consistently, people were able to experience remission. There are also many people I couldn't turn down in joining the course who hadn't done chemotherapy. They ended up never needing chemotherapy or radiation, and they went into remission. I commonly saw tumors shrink in a matter of four weeks. What I was recommending to people in that particular program was using some Chinese herbs to strengthen the immune system, along with very relaxing exercises that would oxygenate the cells, and a very strict dietary regime. The diet involved no packaged foods, a vegetarian diet, and no refined sugars.

One of the most discouraging things I heard during that time was that people would go tell their oncologist what they were doing, and the oncologist would say things like: "There's nothing you can do with your diet that's going to affect the outcome of this cancer." And they still say these kinds of things. That is just like somebody saying, "Why don't we just cut out his or her brain and this cancer will get better?" It's such an uneducated point of view. Who could even say something like that? But it was an oncologist trained at a whole methodology of medicine, who knew nothing about how to promote health, that was saying these things. An oncologist doesn't understand how to create health. He or she only knows how to diagnose a disease and give a drug to reduce the symptoms of it. That is how your oncologist has been trained.

Ninety-five percent of them know very, very little about this science of creating health that I'm talking about. So many other people are trained in creating health and do research to teach people how we have the power within ourselves to be healthy. How we think, how we feel, and what we eat matters. What environmental experience we place ourselves in and the quality of our relationships affect our health, too. We need to gain health from asking ourselves, "Are we giving, every day, some sort of meaningful service to the world?"

There are so many people that do achieve remission from cancer through chemotherapy and radiation. If they've achieved success in life prior to having cancer, they'll almost invariably say that they went through a major breakthrough in making lifestyle choices. For example, they'll say, "I used to prioritize money. I used to prioritize success. My life was extremely busy, but now I see a sunset. Now, I see a little child. I rejoice in that." It's the simple things of life that we're here to do: To be of service to others. To give and receive love. These people wake up and they're grateful for their cancer, which causes them to say, "Stop. You are not living a life you're meant to live." It helps them to discover what we're here for, and that is a major gift that cancer gives to people. That is also part of the process of healing cancer, which is to see any illness, this particular illness, as a gift. Like a yellow light saying, "Slow down, or you're going to miss out what you're here for."

There are a variety of different approaches that are available for people based upon where their heart goes. It can be that they go with their doctors and do their chemotherapy and radiation. Along with that, they may follow programs that will assist their bodies in detoxifying all of the toxins that are already in the body, plus the toxins that were put in the body through chemotherapy. Chemo is a poison that kills, and we want to help the body remove that.

Whether you chose to go the more conventional way or not, there are programs that involve juice fasting. Just drinking eight glasses a day of carrot juice or apple juice, plus eating an apple, carrots, and a few other green vegetables to get lots of minerals, will help. You will need to be drinking throughout the day and not eating many solid foods, except some raw foods. That's one program that's a 5,000 year-old system from Ayurveda. I studied health systems in India and this one is the cancer treatment. Their treatment does not even include an apple; it's just straight carrot juice. It's a carrot juice fast for three months that will treat cancer. I've seen tumors go down in four weeks doing that sort of thing.

Then, there are other groups that come from Germany who took the Indian ideas of Ayurveda and adapted them to more of a raw food diet. This diet involved adding other minerals and a few mineral supplements as well, along with the carrot juice every day. Also, I have a program that involves just removing packaged food from the diet and using lemon. Lemon-fasts include lemonade made from just lemon and water and a little bit of glucose, plus mineral supplements. Another program requires just going on a two-day fast and eating raw foods for a few days. Two-day fasts will help detoxify the body. What happens when you take lemon? Lemon goes into the liver and produces bile to remove those toxins. When the toxins get released out of the liver, the liver can purify the blood better. Your body becomes automatically more alkaline, less acidic.

Another program I am very excited about holds tremendous promise for people who want to go the conventional route for healing faster, healing better and making sure the cancer doesn't come back. This involves whatever approach of cleansing they want to use, dietary adjustments, and using positive imagery along with daily uses of hydrotherapy. This is the oldest treatment in the world for anything. Help your body treat anything through using regular Jacuzzi jets. Get in water - hot water, as hot as you can comfortably stand, about 101 degrees - and you spend about an hour in the bathtub with the jets on. What that does is increase your circulation. That's what warmth does; it increases your circulation, which increases the oxygenation of your cells. Your body sweats in the water and the sweating pulls out the toxins. This is probably one of the most powerful detoxifiers on the planet, as far as when you look at the history of this approach.

The problem is that when people do hydrotherapy, the water is so toxic that within fifteen minutes their fingers will actually start to prune up. This is a sign that your body is becoming dehydrated, rather un-hydrated. Water inside the body flushes toxins in bath water out, so you don't get the effects. But there are new technologies that will super-purify the bath water. You run it through lots of filters. The water is really pure, so your fingers don't prune up.

Also, you can oxygenate the water and that will restore it back to its natural state. When water is in its natural state of purity, your fingers don't prune up. That's how you know you're going to get the optimal results.

So, any person who has cancer - if you're going a conventional route, which statistically has helped many, many people - it may not work for a long period of time. You'll eliminate the problem now, but will it come back? The chances are it will come back, unless you, at this point - when you're the most motivated - decide to make the lifestyle changes needed. You want to no longer continue to create that foundation which gives rise to cancer. Use this wake-up call to motivate yourself to make the choices you need to make. This way, once you can go into remission, you can stay in remission and live a long and healthy life.

Having guided many people through the whole cancer process, working with the alternative systems and the more conventional systems, it's important for people to know that their oncologist can only give them answers that are based upon the worst possible outcome. Oncologists have to protect themselves legally. If they don't tell you the worst possible outcome, you could come back and sue them. So, you're actually going to somebody and asking for advice from somebody who is going to focus on the very worst thing that can happen. They focus on this, rather than the positive, possible things that can happen. So, just keep that in mind.

Your approach, regardless of whether you go with basic, traditional treatment, can be taking the middle of the road and being very safe. I like to help people recognize this. Here you are going to this treatment that's going to help remove these symptoms for a while, so it's giving you some breathing space to take responsibility for solving this problem within yourself. Use this as the wake-up call to motivate you to make healthy changes, too, so that you don't have to be another statistic. For many, after five years, the cancer may come back. This is a statistical time frame, five years, and it commonly happens. Cancer comes back except to those - and I know many - who have taken this time to suddenly make positive choices in their lifestyle. And, the cancer has not come back and it's now been twenty or twenty five years.

As we begin to understand the foundation of cancer and the growth of cancer in the body, it can only grow in the absence of oxygen. Another most important thing for oxygenating ourselves is exercise, but people have a completely wrong idea about exercise. They think that if they exercise hard that they're going to oxygenate their cells more. If they're puffing, they must be getting more oxygen to their cells. But, if you're actually puffing, you're getting less oxygen to your cells, and that's why you're having to breath heavy. You're out of breath, which means you're not getting enough oxygen. So, what you want is the kind of regular exercise that causes you to breathe more deeply but never puts you out of breath. And, people think for good health you've got to feel the burn. Well, the burn is the production of lactic acid. Keep in mind that too much lactic acid causes the body to become too acidic. You don't need to get to the burn if you want to stay healthy. Particularly if you've already been diagnosed with cancer, the last thing you want to be doing is producing more lactic acid.

The very best way to oxygenate your cells is walking - and not just upstairs and not just five minutes, but an hour to two to three hours a day. What you want to do is walk for several hours in the beginning, pretty much on level ground, until you can start walking on hills without getting out of breath. You want to make sure you never get out of breath. Exercise should force you to breath a little deeper than usual. That's all you want - deeper than usual and you want it to be over a long period of time, increasing over the weeks and months, so you're increasing your exercise time. As you do that challenge, your body - in that very easy but challenged way - will grow more capillaries. The growth of capillaries means more oxygen is being delivered to the cells in your body. That's the whole key here. Walking in nature is a very powerful way to oxygenate the cells. Walking by the ocean is another very powerful oxygenator of the cells. Walking in forests, redwood forests in particular is another great oxygenator of the cells. Trees put out a lot of oxygen in the redwood forest.

Another basic thing that people should know when they get sick with cancer is that roses put out a massive amount of oxygen. Fragrant flowers put out a massive amount of oxygen. So you always want to have fresh flowers in your room and in your house when you're sick. Freshness, it's all about oxygenation, will help your body to get better.

There's an old Chinese saying, a 5,000-year-old saying, which is: When nothing else works and one has cancer, the solution is to repose downwind from a rose garden. To repose means to lie and relax, meaning the oxygen from the roses can come to you.

One of the techniques that I would work with in my cancer groups was actually a rose meditation. You would go into a deep relaxed meditation in the presence of a lot of roses, and that would then help oxygenate the cells of the body as well. These are some of those old-fashioned remedies that have great wisdom to them. You can measure just putting a little rose oil on your body, on your toe. Put some rose oil on your toe and measure your oxygen levels in your blood; they'll dramatically go up in one minute. That's how powerful flowers are. It's one of the oldest healing forms on the planet.

We're all being exposed to toxins, and this is certainly so if you're living in the city. You're going to be more exposed to toxic air, and your chances of oxygenating your cells dramatically go down. You can't oxygenate your cells if you're not getting enough oxygen. For example, a hundred years ago, there used to be thirty three percent oxygen in the air. You can look at arctic samples going back thousands of years. If you measure the water in the frozen ice, you know how much oxygen was in the air. It used to be thirty three percent. Today, out in the country, in the woods, it's twenty three percent. If you go into a city, its seventeen or eighteen percent. If you go on a bad day in Tokyo, it's seven percent. At five percent you would die, so oxygenation is a really important thing.

But, I won't say it's all just about having more oxygen in the air, although that's certainly going to help. Your body has to be able to absorb oxygen as well. You could have all the oxygen in the world outside of you, but if your body is acidic, you can't absorb it. As you detoxify the acids and you become more alkaline in your body, if you're still not exposing yourself to the fresh oxygen, you won't have enough in order to help the body heal and stay healthy. Pollution has a huge impact on the amount of oxygen that gets to the cells. Pollution has a direct impact on the potential of cancer.

http://www.marsvenus.com/

Bernie Siegel, M.D.

Surgeon
Author

I became a surgeon for healthy reasons. I went into medicine because I like people and care about them. I wanted to help them. I was an artist as a child, so I was very good with my hands. When I sat down and thought it out, I thought: "You're good with your hands, you like to fix things, you like people, you like science. Become a doctor, become a surgeon. It will put everything together for you."

In medical school, nobody deals with the fact that you have to take care of people as well as what you're going to feel. Because then, you realize you can't fix everything. It's not like working on a piece of wire or plumbing. This is a human being and they die. They have things you can't cure, and never in medical school - or anywhere - does anybody sit you down and say, "How are you going to deal with this? How are you going to feel when your patient dies?" Or, you may make a mistake in the operating room. Even if it's a malpractice situation, you're human; you can't fix every damn thing.

Out of that pain, I started going to workshops, which I give myself credit for. To deal with my stuff, my feelings - which was the day that transformed my life - I was sitting in this workshop when one of my patients plops down next to me. There's no desk now to save my life and keep us apart. She said, "You're a nice guy, I feel better when I'm in the office with you, but I can't take you home with me, so I need to know how to live between office visits." She was there, and I was there. I always say, "MD stands for my disease." We were both there for our wounds and health. But when she said that I thought, "Wow, I can stop feeling like a failure. I don't have to have pain all the time; I can help people live, instead of trying to keep people from being dead." Believe me, I even thought of going into veterinary medicine so I wouldn't have all the pain. One day I told one of my patients, who was a vet, what I wanted to do. He said, "Don't, because it's people that bring the pets in." He made it obvious to me that the problem is helping people, not finding another job.

So I started support groups back in 19... I think the first one met in 1978. And this again was my wake up call. I sent a hundred letters to patients from our office who had cancer and the letter said, "We're starting a group to help you live a longer, better life - come on." I went out and I read a lot of books, and I learned a lot of things on how to help patients and how to help them survive. I forgot to put at the bottom that this was only for the people in our office; you can't bring friends and relatives. I mailed it and I thought, "Oh my, they're going to bring all their friends and relatives and you'll have five hundred people show up. What are you going to do with them?" I really was in a panic for weeks. Then, at the first meeting, less than a dozen women showed up. I thought, "I don't know the people I'm taking care of. I'm offering them a longer, better life and nobody shows up." And that woke me up, too. I needed to know what they were living in their experiences, and that's very much what I try to treat now. I'm not doing the surgery anymore, but it doesn't matter. You can help people with words, because one thing - I don't know where I first saw it - if you write the word "words" continuously, with no space, it becomes "swords." I thought, "Wow, you can kill or cure with words, or you can kill or cure with a scalpel."

We sat down and we talked, and I began to see if you help people live, they will out do statistics. Some literally had a miraculous healing, their disease disappeared. Now I call it "as they rebirth themselves," become born again. They each became a new person. It was amazing what happened.

I began to write books accidentally. People said, "Do you ever think of writing down all this stuff?" I said, "If you want to help me, fine," so we ended up writing a book. As an artist, the worst grade I got in college was in creative writing, so I was not a writer. What I did was just talk about it, and then somebody typed it out, and a book came. That's when I got into all the famous talk shows because I was obviously a problem. I was telling people their life had something to do with their disease, so I was blaming them. That was the interpretation. You're telling them it's their fault and they're to blame. We were on all the famous talk shows. I wish I could go back and be on those shows then with what I know today. Because I was busy trying to make it scientific, defend myself, show them how this affects.... and what you got into was conflict. I finally began to realize I should just tell stories and stop fighting with people and arguing. The stories will get through.

First, I wouldn't talk like a scientist. If doctors were arguing with me, I would say things like, "Did you read this journal? Did you see this?" I would say, "This article was even in the New York Times." The doctor might say to me, "That's not a medical journal." He can't accept what I'm saying. "Oh, the New York Times, we don't have to count that." It was just ridiculous. I was really arguing with the fact that they couldn't accept what I was saying, even if it was a fact. They didn't want to accept it. If I had to do it again today, as I said, I would stick with the stories, not try to be statistical. Not try to validate anything, just tell stories so they could walk out saying, "Well, he just told us case history or anecdotes." So they're not mad at me, and we're not yelling at each other. And, what they'll do is go home, something will come into their office, and they'll say, "Hey, that's what he was talking about, I'll give him a ring. Or, I'll send him a note." This way, we'd begin to dialog. Then, you could begin to talk about the medical literature and what has been said.

This psychiatrist called Maninger.....when I wrote my book and sent it to him to read, he wrote back saying: "I was about to write a book called "Twelve Hopeless Cases", about twelve people with incurable diseases who are all well today. But I don't have to because you just wrote it." What I learned was when I sent articles to medical journals, they came back saying, "This is interesting, but it's totally inappropriate." When I sent to ones who were appropriate - meaning psychotherapy, psychology journals - it came back again saying, "Yes, it's appropriate, but it's not interesting. We know this." That's when I began to see how chopped up medicine is. I say, if you're a plumber or electrician you don't read the other guy's journal. So, if you're a surgeon or an oncologist, you don't read what the psychiatrist is reading. They may see things in their practice that you don't see, or become aware of.

Because I was sitting in groups with people, I was really in both worlds. Even some of the oncologists in town criticized me. They said, "You're not a psychiatrist, you

don't know what the hell you're doing. You shouldn't be..."
I said, "What are you mad at me for? I'm trying to help
people." I said, "I may not help them, but I won't hurt
them." But they were enraged. However, that same group
of oncologists became my best supporters. Because I began
to send them the patients, who my wife labeled "the
exceptional patients" who were willing to talk about
feelings, look at their lives, make changes. As I sent them
there, see, that's what changed the doctors They began to
notice - these people are different. Some of them don't die
when they are supposed to. Some of them have their
disease disappear, even though we know the treatment isn't
any good.

One anecdote - my father-in-law was quadriplegic due to
an accident - so he had people coming to his home to care
for him. One of them got a phone call from her cousin in
North Carolina. What's the call? "I've got cancer. The
doctor said to not even bother to go to Duke. Why drive
for several hours to get chemotherapy, which will make you
feel worse? You're going to die of the disease anyway, so go
home and just enjoy the last few months." The woman says
to her cousin, "Dr. Siegel makes people well all the time,
get up here." She shows up. I don't even know about this
and I get a phone call. "My cousin's here with cancer." I
said, "Well, I'll admit her to the hospital."

I admit her, go into see her, and it turns out she has
leukemia, which is nothing to do with surgery. But, I sat
down on the bed. I talked to her. I told her we'd get people
in to see her and so forth. The oncologist from this group
sees her and says to me, "There isn't much we can do for
her. I mean, the chemotherapy is not very effective. We'll
give her something, and we'll try and do something for

her." And then I start getting letters from him about how well she's doing, how remarkable her response is - and finally a letter a few months later - no sign of leukemia. Then, with a smile, "Isn't chemotherapy wonderful?" Because he knew this had nothing to do with what he was doing. I said to her cousin who was up here, "She's had this remarkable result." And she said, "I know why," and I said, "Why?" She said, "My cousin told me that when you sat on her bed and hugged her, she knew she'd get better." When she went home, I got letters saying, "I'm driving my doctor crazy because I walk down the street, and when I see him, I make sure I cross over and walk right up to him. He doesn't know what to do with me, because I'm supposed to be dead."

But when I saw things like that, I realized there's nothing wrong...see this was another argument you get into on television with giving people hope, and they would say, "You're giving false hope." You can't give false hope, you know. I can hope I'm going to win the lottery. Now, if I'm an idiot and go out and spend hundreds and thousands of dollars knowing I'm going to win the lottery, that's different. I mean, that's stupidity, that's not hope. But if I buy a lottery ticket, fine. I may feel good for a week thinking, "I could win and if I don't, I don't," But what I found is that, yes, when you give people hope, it improves their lives, and nobody's ever mad at you for bringing hope and love and laughter into their life. They don't say, " I died anyway. What was the point?"

Another doctor in Chicago said he noticed that people that came further than fifteen miles had three times as frequent a response to his treatment than people who lived near the hospital. Again, you begin to see, there's something in the person. The quantum physicist states that "desire and intention alter the physical world, because things occur that would not normally occur if they were not desired." The people who have a will to live, do better. But saying, "If I didn't cure myself, then I didn't love enough, or change my life enough," I see this too. They grow up with guilt and blame and shame and this is partially why I recently wrote my last book on parenting. You say, "What does that have to do with anything?" Besides my being the father of five children, which taught me a lot, I learned from listening to people in the support groups and what their parents did to them.

And one statistic out of Harvard showed that while you were at Harvard, if you were asked, "Did your parents love you?" in this survey the students who said, "Yes, my parents loved me," thirty five years later, approximately one out of four had suffered a major illness. Those who said, "My parents didn't love me," 98% had suffered a major illness. So you begin again to see that your diet, your exercise, your mental attitude - a whole host of things, addictions - all these things were related to health. Was I loved? Am I worth something? That's why I talk about re-parenting and re-birthing people, and some of the wonderful poems I have. So, if you see life as a labor pain, that's another aspect.

Going through surgery, chemotherapy, radiation or whatever is not a big problem. You have far fewer side effects because you're saying this is worth it. One woman compared nine months of giving birth to her child to the twelve months of treatment. If you give birth yourself, it's worth it. But, if the physician inflicts it on you, then you are going to have far more side effects. What they saw in one study in New York was that when people got into their car and started driving to the hospital, their white count went down - and they haven't even gotten there yet. How powerful your mind is imagining it. That's why I do a lot of work with drawings. If you said, "I'm going to have surgery next week, do you think it's the right thing to do? I wouldn't sit down and intellectually discuss it with you; I would say, "Draw a picture of yourself in the operating room."

For some it's hell. I mean the devil could be cutting you up. Others show God over the operating room with this beautiful spiritual symbol and the surgeon holding you. You know, they're going to wake up and do very well, because they see this as a gift that is going to cure them and make them well versus being cut up and mutilated. This is something that most doctors are not trained to understand. What I call separating your head from your heart. You need surgery. Well, you should say, "Why don't you ask me how I feel about it? Or, ask me how I feel about you as my surgeon or anything else."

Particularly, when you do children's surgery...kids who are not loved really feel that their parents are bringing them here to be cut up and punished. When you say to these kids, "Here's a bunch of crayons," they'll picture the operating room. They'll pick up the black and red. It's a horror scene. And the kids who are loved pick up the blues and greens; it's just this beautiful peaceful picture because they know this is not a punishment, but a way to make them feel better.

I always say to people, "What are you experiencing?" Not, "What is your diagnosis?" but "What does it mean to you? How does it feel to hear this?" The words that pop out of people, I then relate back to their life. If they say "blockage," "wake-up call," "draining," "burden," whatever words pop out, I say, "What else fits?" That way, we help heal their lives. If you eliminate all the burdens in your life, you'll feel better and healthier. The other thing is, I try to get them to understand that you don't die based on statistics. I mean, some people do. The doctor says there's no hope for you, boom, you go home, get in bed and lie down and die. But you're not a statistic, so I try to teach what I call survival behavior. What are the qualities of people who outdo the statistics and the expectations? I approach it in a sense, again, that if you were an athlete or an actor, you have to rehearse and practice. So, let's start doing that. You don't become critical of yourself if you miss a line in a play or don't make a touch down on every play. It's okay. Let me try again. Let's see what we can get right.

And just as I said, using the terms "re-birthing" and "born again." What you're doing is acting as if you're the person you want to be. We give you a role model. If you're a survivor, this is how you would behave. It's expressing feelings, saying no to things you don't want to do. Asking for help. There's literally a list of questions that you would present to people. Not living a role, but living an authentic life. Because, many people literally give up their lives to make everybody else happy. So if you learn you have six months to live, then why go to a job you hate or be in a marriage that's killing you? It's helping people to redefine themselves.

Recently, what I read was about a gentleman who had several friends die of AIDS. This man was told he was HIV positive, because a doctor got a report back. They repeated the test, and it came back negative. It turns out the first test had a mistake in the report. But nobody told him. He literally went home, got into bed, and developed every symptom that he'd seen his friends have. He was close to dying when the doctor was reviewing a whole bunch of patients, saw the computer printout, and looked at his. The doctor realized he was negative. They went and told him. Within two weeks, the man was well again.

Now, the other side of the coin. I would get letters from people who were HIV positive, even in prisons. That's the part that impressed me. It was the person changing. They couldn't get out of prison, but they changed their attitude toward life. Another who said that when you live in your heart, magic happens. But, doctors would say, "Oh, your first test must have been a mistake," or "You've had a miracle." This woman in prison said to the doctor, "It's a miracle. My blood tests were not all mistakes." It was the same message that if I have a belief, if I'm willing to do things, things change. Because, what people have to realize is, this is all science. You're changing your body chemistry.

I was giving a lecture at an office where one of our son's works. They had a health week for all employees, and he brought one of his kids. So I said to this group of adults, "What day of the week is bad for your health?" And Sam screams, "Saturday!!" His father starts saying, "Sssshh!" because he knows that's the wrong answer. I said, "Wonderful, Sam, that's exactly the point I'm trying to make." When I go into schools, talking to third, fourth, and fifth-graders, I say, "What day of the week is bad for your health?" The kids yell, "Saturday and Sunday!!" At first, I said, "Saturday and Sunday are bad for your health?" and the kids said, "Yes, we get so tired running around doing all the things we love to do, we're exhausted." Right, you're doing what you love to do, but what do adults answer? "Monday, because I have to go to work." So, we have more heart attacks, suicides, strokes and illnesses on Monday mornings. It's very obvious you can't separate your chemistry from your life. And when you are feeling good, it's very different.

There's a book out by Bruce Lipton, The Biology of Belief. It has to do, again, with some of what I've talked about with parenting. Up to the age of six, a child's brain wave patterns are like that of somebody hypnotized. So if you get negative messages, you have a real struggle getting rid of them when you become conscious and aware. But the other point the author was making is: If you're under stress and fear, that's a coping mechanism built into us to protect us. If I'm sitting here and a rabid dog runs in, yes, stress and fear are wonderful, because I'm going to jump up and get the hell out of here faster than I've ever moved before in my life. Or, I'll be able to jump up on a piece of furniture and be able to save myself. But, if I feel threatened every time I go everywhere, like from my disease, then my stress hormone level goes up, my immune function goes down. The blood is not going to my brain or organs that need it, but to muscles to get me out of here. That's the part that people have to understand. So if they're living with this negative, stressful image, they're making themselves more vulnerable. If they switch into love, then, it's growth, and I mean that literally. If you're massaged, loved, touched - this helps. You see this with infants and orphans, who used to die in the 1800s because people didn't touch them. We were afraid that we're infecting them. No, they're getting infected because nobody is giving them any love or attention or touch. So when you get a massage, when you get a hug and share love, you're making yourself, in a sense, invulnerable to diseases that other people may pick up - whether it's the flu or anything else. When you're doing what you love, you're also more resistant to disease.

One of my bumper stickers is "Eat Well, Exercise and Die Anyway." I say to people, "I'm not trying to keep you from being dead; I'm trying to get you to enjoy life."

I'll say to people, "I've twin sisters. One is a sweet little girl who makes mommy and daddy happy and never expresses anger; the other's a little devil who has no trouble expressing her feelings. Who's more likely to get breast cancer?" And, of course everybody votes for the good girl, and it's true. So again, if you're not expressing your feelings, what are you doing to yourself? And that's the hard part. When people use love, which I tell them to do, as a weapon, this works. When people are driving you crazy, love them. I mean, it's an age-old message. See that's the part I also look for. What are the themes I can find, you might say, in Buddhism, the Bible, Talmud? It doesn't matter where you look. What is the advice they're giving to people to survive? It's exactly the same message over the centuries, you know, to "love thy neighbor as thyself," because you gotta love yourself. Bring forth what is within you. If not, it will destroy you, and it goes on and on and on. I see these common themes. He who seeks to save his life will lose it....If you give up your life to make everybody happy, you've lost your life.

How do you save your life? By eliminating what's killing you. That's the part I try to get across to kids. I say, "Don't kill yourself; eliminate what's killing you." Because they don't understand, because they are not living their life. It's imposed by Mom and Dad, what they want me to be, so what am I am going to do? And I think when we reclaim our lives, and start saying yes to ourselves and no to what we don't want to do, then a lot of healing occurs.

One thing I've been reading is that people who take their aggression and turn it into work or play, will remain healthy. Think about football players. Sometimes, they get violent on the field, through banging heads and knocking people down. But meet them, as I have, off the field. They're the sweetest, calmest people. They're getting aggression out on the field. Or, put it into work. I'm building things and I'm banging away. Fine, you don't go home angry and beat your family up. Most people don't know how to get their aggression out in a healthy way. Look at our society. We're killing each other over religions and nationalities, races. It's ridiculous.

My solutions, even for the world's problems, would be why don't we use the money to build something? Martin Luther King was saying the same thing. Spend billions, not on wars, but on helping people - what a different world you'd have. Because it's hard for people to be aggressive when you say, "I love you" to them. I mean this literally. People don't know how to handle love. The fact that we grow up fearful and with poor images of ourselves leads us to hurt others as well. When I get criticized, that used to be hard for me, because I'm out trying to help people. They'll come up and say, "Well, I heard your talks before, and you just said the same thing. I'm sorry I came. I don't agree with you. You made me feel worse." I would go home and think, "Boy, I gotta do it better next time." But I began to realize the next person in line might say, "That was wonderful and inspiring. Thank you."

What you begin to realize is that people project what's in them onto you. So, when I get critical letters, emails now, I say to people, "I love you, sorry your parents didn't." I don't try to justify what I said and tell them that I was right. I don't get into arguments; I just say, "I love you." And I think that's a big part of the problem in the world today. If we grew up loved, we would see that in others too. Something to love in another person, and we would connect very differently. But when you grew up with resentments and anger and hatred and all kinds of things within you, then that's what gets projected on other people. When they say something, or do something, yes, you're very critical of them. They're sinners, terrible. It's amazing what people write to me because I misquote somebody or do some little thing. They say how terrible I am.

People can choose to love. You have AIDS, cancer, your home burns down, whatever it is, and then you say, "Now I realize what's important about life." If we grew up with that.... So, I think parents, teachers and clergy are the ones who could really save the world. In my latest book I put a poem in which a woman said that in kindergarten she drew a picture and the teacher came over and criticized it. This was because she made a purple tent, and the teacher said tents aren't purple - that's a spiritual color.

In first grade the teacher said we're going to draw a picture. Here's paper and crayons, she said. I left the page blank. The teacher walked over, put his hand on my head, and said how beautiful and bright the snowfall was. What a difference, you see.

If we let the person know that "I love you. I may not like what you have done, but I'm not saying there's something wrong with you." So, you feel loved and then your approach to life is very different. I teach people using my sense of humor. I'm always saying after reading something by a Rabbi: When you read at the beginning of the Bible, it says everything God created was good, but when God created man, you don't see that in the next sentence. He said the Hebrew word "Tov' should be interpreted as "complete," because the word "good" is used too frequently without having any real meaning. He said, "If you think about it, everything God created was complete, except man."

Yeah, when you say to some people, "What is it like to experience cancer?" they say, "Wake-up call, blessing, new beginning," and they become more complete.

What you need is your role model. My role model is saying, " WWLD (What Would Lassie Do?). What should I do?" Whenever I have a problem, I say, "What would Lassie do?" and then I go do it.

In many ways the animals are wonderful teachers, in terms of love, forgiveness, a whole host of things. You know it's interesting when I think about love and things regarding the computer and email. I get more photographs sent to me of animals loving each other. I never get twelve pictures of people doing beautiful things. Like this morning, there are dogs licking cats, kittens and polar bears sticking their heads in the window, rubbing noses with the photographer. I mean, look, sleeping together. All these creatures and you'd say, "What is going on here?"

Our house has always been filled with animals, and I felt that gave our kids reverence for life. They really care about life. They'll carry insects out of the house instead of swatting them. What a difference they make in the world because of the fact that they were brought up with a reverence for life. I think there are many teachers out there for us.

When people say, "I'm afraid," I ask for a better definition. What are you afraid of? What does that mean? And they say, "I'm afraid of dying," and I say I don't know what that means either. What do you mean, you're afraid of dying? Because very honestly, I think being dead is a hell of a lot easier than being alive. I've had a near-death experience as a child, almost choked to death, left my body. I didn't want to come back, and I mean that literally. I mean I was mad as hell when I didn't die. This may sound crazy to people, but I was very angry that I wasn't allowed to die - which I wanted to do - because it was a lot more interesting out there than in here. I mean, past lives, a whole host of things, but I think consciousness goes on. Let's put it that way. What we've learned in this life goes on.

But when you say, "I'm afraid of dying," what do you mean? People get into "I may be alone, I may be in pain." Let's sit down and decide how we're going to solve that. Is there somebody in your family you can talk to? Let's sit down with the doctors, so if you have pain, you'll speak up and get the right treatment. Because that's also the appropriate anger I try to teach people. If you're not treated with respect in the hospital, speak up. In the top ten causes of death is "being hospitalized due to medical errors." Those are the nice patients. They're submissive sufferers who don't make any noise. This is all part of survival behavior. But usually, when you define the fears, people begin to realize: Okay, I have some power to take care of that. If you get to the point you don't want to keep living, that's okay too. What's interesting to me is that I was really impressed with how easy it was for people to die, if they had made the choice to live.

In other words, in going through things, if they had families that loved them and supported them, when they said, "I'm tired," they left. I've watched my parents and in-laws have no trouble dying, and I mean that literally. My father-in-law, as I mentioned, was quadriplegic. One night, when he was in his nineties - he was a really brave guy that I admired - I said to him, "Why don't you live to be 100, so we can get you on television? Let the world see you." He let me know that he was not going to live to 100 because his son-in-law wanted him to, in terms of what he was going through. He was 97 at the time with his wife, daughter, and myself feeding him dinner and giving him his vitamins. He just shook his head no and didn't open his mouth. He was saying, "No, I'm done. I'm tired." He died that night.

You'd say, "How did he manage? He wasn't dying at that moment." But that's something I learned and saw in all our family members. In the hospital, most people die in the middle of the night. Why? Because the family isn't there to make you feel guilty, and the doctors aren't there to stop you.

As physicians, death is failure. You're failing, and so we will run in and try to keep you alive two more days. People realize: I gotta get out of here, when the doctor isn't around. I found when I help people to live, they had a lot less trouble dying, and they can die surrounded by loved ones. My father literally died laughing because of the stories my mother was telling - surrounded by everybody in the family who loved him. Those are the things I share in some of my books. But, that also helped me empower people. To get back to that geneticist Bruce Lipton, he was talking about the fact that genes don't decide what's going to happen. They get a signal. That's why identical twins, the longer they live, the more differences there are in their genetic makeup. This is also why they don't get the same disease on the same day - because of the separate lives they are living.

So, I can have a gene that never gets turned on and never get a disease that my twin gets. Why? Because I'm enjoying life and he isn't. It gets back to what messages are you giving your body? Is it a "live" message, or are you living in fear? I've seen people die when the doctor said, "Well, you have cancer of the lung. I also know you have cataracts, but there's no point in taking out your cataracts because you're going to be dead in a few months. The health plan is not going to pay for your cataract surgery." That guy died in six days, and his family sued the health planner and I was behind them all the way. Because I think that what that doctor said killed him.

If we can train doctors in how to talk, you would have far fewer people having side effects. It's like watching the commercials on TV after you hear about a drug. The last thirty seconds, they tell you a hundred and twelve things that could go wrong if you take it. When you're in a doctor's office, they don't rush that. They say, "Here, read this list." I put this in one of my books about the chemotherapy agent Adriamycin. You're handed a list of all the side effects of Adriamycin. There's nothing on this whole page that says this is good for you, such as it could make your cancer shrink, go away, you'll feel better. Everything on the page is what will go wrong. We know from studies that if you go in, get an injection of saline, and you're told it's chemotherapy, your hair falls out.

You get a drug to grow hair, with some receiving a placebo as a control. Their hair grows. This works with depression, too. Placebos work just as well as some of the anti-depressants. So, what people believe has a lot to do with outcomes. Years ago, they even did surgery on people with heart problems. They would make an incision and sew it up, and they had a dramatic improvement. Lots of people thought their heart was repaired.

So what goes on in your mind obviously manifests itself in your body. And it's becoming more scientific to prove. That's why I don't get on all the talk shows with people yelling at me now.

If you get back to AIDS, cancer - it doesn't matter which. The optimistic volunteers do better statistically in terms of survival than those who are saying, "No, I'm a victim. Why is God punishing me?" That's why I also get back to religion.

It blew my mind to listen to people feeling that they deserved a disease. I'm guilty, I did this, God is punishing me. And what I try to tell people, and why I started to study religions, is that some religions are healthy and some are unhealthy in terms of the burden they put on you. But I will say to people, "If you lose your car keys, does God want you to walk home?" And they laugh and they say no, and I say, "What do you do?" and they reply, "I look for my keys." Fine, if you lose your health, go look for that. That message came from Maimonides, the Jewish physician, I think about eight or nine hundred years ago. He said if we find what our neighbor has lost, we restore it to our neighbor. And health is the same thing. So if people look at it as if they've lost something, saying "I'm not being punished, nothing is being taken from me, this is better. They should not say, "What did I do wrong?" They should say, "Let me find what I've lost." Then they may set out on that journey.

The craziness of medicine… in an oncology journal they were discussing malignant melanomas and how women live longer than men with the same stage. And this oncologist wrote in the journal: "It must be something to do with female hormones protecting them." I read this and I laughed. Because my comment is: Married men live longer than single men with the same disease, so is sleeping with female hormones helping them? People laugh when you say that. Women have connections, relationships. It's not saying, "I can't work. What's the point of living?" But the women, you know, say, "I can't die until I'm married and out of the house," and on and on. But I also try to get the women not to live a role. Not to be Mama. Because I've seen cancer come back after many years, when all the kids left home. And that, again, as a doctor, always blew my mind. How did you keep it under control while you're a Mama? Recently, I even had a letter from the child of the woman who developed breast cancer while pregnant, but she did not give up the child. The woman had surgery, but refused other treatment to give birth. This was an incredible, wonderful woman. The letter to me ended with this: "Cancer made me take a look at myself, and I like who I met."

And here we are, twenty years later getting a letter from her child saying, "Thank you, for what you did with my mother and what my mother taught us." The woman ultimately did die of cancer, but it was a gift to the kid to know how to survive. I also say to people, "You want to be

44

immortal? Love somebody. It's the only way to be immortal." When you start living your life, then you reap the benefits.

As a father of five, I can tell you who gets your attention. It's the kid who's driving you nuts. But who asks you, "How come you don't love me?" The kid who's an angel. I had to explain to him that I'm not paying as much attention to him because his brother is driving me crazy. But he really asked me, "Why don't I get as much time as everybody else?" If you give them that love, they end up very differently.

One more thing than popped into my head about men. What's interesting is that even to get them to come to the group to share that feeling and the love and experience, it is difficult. We can give you the love and let you know we care about you. But when the husband has cancer, the wives always show up. When the wife has cancer, it's a damn rare guy who's willing to come in the room and sit there. When you go around the room and say, "Why are you here?" the husbands would always say, "I'm her chauffeur." That way, I don't have to say a damn thing, I just drove her here. One of them wrote a wonderful poem called "The Chauffeur" that I put into another one of my books. What he shared with readers was sharing the journey. There may be a glass partition, but we're sharing and he's trying to help his wife get to where she's going. It was a wonderful way of turning it into something meaningful.

The feminine qualities are the survival qualities. So when you can get the men to get into relationships and connections - and not just asking what can I do? - they are far more likely to survive.

One commercial airline pilot said something interesting, I was talking about fear before, because he came to the cancer group and said, "I was taught how to deal with fear. When you're up in the air, five miles up in the air and the engine goes out, what do you do? You announce to everybody, 'Don't worry, folks, we have another engine.' But that one goes out, what do you do? You announce to everyone, 'Don't worry folks, we'll find a nice place to land.' But what if you're over the ocean? 'Don't worry folks, we'll find a ship and come down next to the ship.' But I don't see any ship. 'Don't worry, we'll find a nice soft wave, and come down next to that." You know, he had this whole routine, so when somebody said, "You have cancer?" the answer is, "Okay, now let's find a place where we can land, and let's see what we can do about it."

That's why I say how important parenting is. I used to say at workshops, "What models do you live by?" Because of my parents, I grew up with things like, "do what makes you happy", so you pay attention to your feelings. When you had troubles, "God was re-directing you, something good will come of this". You grow up with that and it's hard to have anything go wrong. People would come up to me and say, "You're not asking what models we're dying by." If you grew up with: "We can't be proud of you, you embarrass us all the time," and "you can only wear black, brown or navy blue because we don't want people to notice you," - it's hard. And her quote was: "My mother's words were eating away at me and it maybe gave me cancer." When she got cancer, she bought a red dress. She was red from the shoes to the top of her head. But when she handed me this two-page letter about her life, I thought, "How wonderful." You can see her from a mile away, but she reclaimed her life. It's a big part of why she's still walking around today, that she didn't live her mother's limits.

When I was in airports, I'd meet these kids with green hair, piercings - so bazaar. I always go and sit down next to them and say, "How come you're trying to be inconspicuous?" They always burst out laughing, and we talk. A lot of them are like that because they don't want anybody near them. They've been hurt.

One woman came into my office. She'd had surgery on her upper thigh for cancer. The plastic surgeon that operated on her called me and said; "I don't know what's wrong with this lady. She keeps screaming how ugly I made her. Nobody even knows she has a scar unless she's in a bathing suit." He asked would I talk to her. So, she came over to the office and I simply said to her, "How do you describe what you're experiencing?" And she said, "Failure." I said, "How does that fit your life?" She said, "My body has failed." I said, "Excuse me, that's not my question. How does failure fit your life?" Then she said, "My parents committed suicide when I was a child, so I must have been a failure as a child." She had decided never to get close to anybody, because she didn't want to get hurt again. And she said, "Oh at work, I know people's names, and that's where it ends." The cancer, in a sense, shook her up and woke her up. She began to change and started to live again. I asked her to draw a picture of herself. It's this rigid masculine picture. But what I did like was, she was all there. People leave parts out but she was standing there like a soldier. All the parts were there. I knew that she had the potential to change. She wasn't missing a head or hands so that she couldn't reach out. She could do it.

There are a lot of side effects to cancer, but they're not all bad. One of the things that keeps me happy is I accept my mortality. That's a good way of explaining it. One example of this is the movie "Harold & Maude," if you've seen that wonderful movie. The more I watch it, because I think it was done twenty years ago, the more I learn from it. That's another thing people need to understand. Keep reading the same books and watching the same movies. If they don't get better, you're stuck. But if they get smarter, you're more aware of things now. Last time I watched that movie, maybe a year ago, something struck me at the end. Here's this boy who's into death. He gets a car and turns it into a hearse. The last scene, you see the hearse go off a cliff. You figure he's committed suicide, because the 80-year-old, played by Ruth Gordon, has died and he's going to kill himself, too. But the last scene, no. He's walking away with his banjo, smiling. I realize he's eliminated death from his life. He's now living.

Two guys were talking and one is talking about black and horrible - and how desolate life is. The first guy goes on and on and on, and the other fellow says, "What are you doing Saturday night?" The first guy says, "I'm committing suicide". But the next line really struck me, the other guy says, "How about Friday night?" I thought, "Okay, you're going to commit suicide Saturday night, why screw up Friday?" That's why I feel very empowered by my mortality. I know damn well I'm going to die - that's not my problem. My problem is how do I feel today? So I don't give my power away. Somebody can insult me, or we've been robbed, things can happen. But, I don't get up every day hanging onto the guy who insulted me, robbed me. I get back to: How can I give love? If somebody in our family is sick, I'm not every day thinking that I can't cure them. It's about how can I love them, and let them know I love them, and just be there to listen to them - even when I can't fix anything. I'm not saying there aren't moments when I get into the doctor's place and they say, "You're not helping me, Dad." You know, giving them advice, it's all about getting back to loving them and stop telling them what to do.

A study was done about a year or so ago at Yale. I try to do a lot of research, because people would say to me, "Have you done research?" "No, I haven't." Well then. When I tried to do research, people would say, "You're nuts. We're not giving you money." Whether it was playing music in the operating room, putting videos in the patient's rooms so they could relax, see things. Every time I tried to do that, I got, "You're experimenting on human beings. Fill out a hundred pages of forms, or we're not going to give you $2,500." Even if I said, "I could save you a million. All the patients would go home sooner," it didn't matter, so I got criticized for not doing research. But, nobody believed in it.

Now they've done the research. Because twenty years, thirty years later, everybody says, "Oh yeah, play music in an operating room. The patients had less anesthetic and had less pain, so they recovered faster and needed fewer drugs." If you played stories for kids and then played it during the surgery, the same thing happened. I saw this when I played the music. Not only did the patients do better, but so did everybody in the operating room. We were all calmer and more relaxed. So, I brought humor in as well as the music - changing the environment to a place to heal - to having people write notes with magic markers on their body for surgeons. When I get letters from people saying - I had the whole operating room laughing - and this is somebody seriously ill with cancer - they are wondering why is her doctor laughing? I mean, she's so ill, why? Because she wrote a note to him on her belly. This humor changes the whole feeling in the operating room.

I tell people to go to the hospital and take a magic marker, a noisemaker and a water gun. Why do you want a magic marker? You can write: Not this one, stupid, cut here. You can use the noisemaker when you don't get a response to the call button. Somebody in our support group would be dead today, if she didn't have a roommate, because she said, "Nobody came and I was choking on food. My roommate ran out and got help and saved me." The water gun was used by a teenager, because he was in the hospital dying. He'd close his door to be with his family and girlfriend. People would come in for a lot of dumb reasons - to clean the room or empty a wastebasket. He'd take out his water gun and drench them. The nurses were smart enough to never take it away from him, because they knew this was his way to deal with anger and let it out. When the nurses and the doctors get sick, they write books because now they're not the tourist. This is interesting, because a woman used these terms in her poem about a native and a tourist.

The tourists are really the healthcare professionals. If you haven't been sick, you're a tourist. You don't know what the natives are doing. When we get sick, we learn a lot. I spent a week in bed in a hospital. I learned a hell of a lot, and I became a much better doctor because I knew what my patients were going through. If I were in charge of medical education, it would be something every healthcare professional would have to do - spend a week in the hospital where they don't know you. Get admitted with some terrible diagnosis and just lie here for a few days. See how you're treated - what it's like to be the patient and the difference that makes.

I feel that we're here to serve. The spiritual message is: "We're not here to be served, but to serve." But how you serve is your decision. If I want to be a doctor, fine. If I want to be a plumber, run a restaurant, that's my choice, but I'm going to help people in my way. Not doing what Mom and Dad say they're going to be proud of. When people haven't lived their lives, then it's hard to die. I see them dying angry, because they never got what they wanted. They wanted love from people and never got it. This is not love: if you're doing it to get paid back, you're doing it for the wrong reasons.

What would I say to someone who has cancer? I would say to them, "You're not a statistic. Even if you have one chance in a hundred or in ten thousand, it doesn't matter. If you have one chance in ten thousand, fine."

Giving another example: There was a medical student, while at Harvard, who developed a brain tumor. After surgery, he was blind and they told him, "I'm sorry, you're going to be dead within a year, and you'll be blind." Well, his sight came back after he left the hospital, so he thought, "Hey, my sight came back, maybe I can live." He said he went to the Harvard Medical Library to read all the books on his type of tumor. He said every single book said recurrence is invariable, death within a year.

And I said to him, "Jordan, if you'd been a good medical student, you would have gone home, gotten in bed, and died." He was a lousy student; he got mad as hell. He said,

"How dare they say 'invariable?'" Now, he went through chemotherapy, he went through radiation. But, he also changed his life, his diet, his attitude, and the tumor never came back. So again, you see, what would I say to someone who came to me and said, "There's no hope?" I'd say, "Let's see what happens. If you want to give it a shot, what've you got to lose?"

You can leave your troubles to God, you can move to Montana where you always wanted to live, you can take your tie off and stop worrying about if you look right. You can get a divorce; you can quit your job. Whatever comes up for that person.

The key word is "responsibility." It's not "blame" or "guilt." My word is not "patient." You have to become a responsible "participant". It's not about blaming yourself - it's participating. I would also say to them, "Draw your home and family, draw yourself, your disease, your treatment, your immune system. Draw an outdoor scene - all these pictures and we'll sit and look at them." In the symbols are the things that I can help them with. If you didn't put arms on, I'd say, "How are you going to reach out for what you need?" If you don't have ears, if you don't have a nose, how do you get inspiration? How do we breathe life into you? If you don't have legs, how the hell are you going to go anywhere or do anything? Or, if I look at their family and they're all over the place. Come on - you want something. Let's get them together and let's help you.

I can help guide them as a therapist in a sense, also. If the treatment looks like hell with this black bottle hanging, I'd say, "We've got to think about this. If you feel this treatment is horror and worse than your disease, maybe you don't want to do this."

The way I put it is this: "Are you trying not to die or trying to do what's right for you?" If you're trying not to die, then do every damn thing that anybody tells you. Then you're not mad at yourself someday. But, if it's what's right for me, what labor pain am I willing to go through to birth myself? Then you don't get mad at yourself. If you don't cure yourself, if it doesn't go away, okay. This is my decision, I've tried. It's to empower the patient. I know people who are literally driven to the cemetery by their family members who say, "We don't want you here, so you go and do this treatment." If my family did that, I'd say, "You do the treatment first and tell me if you still want me to do it."

That's why you say to people, "What would you do if you had fifteen minutes to live?" And my reaction would be to pick up the phone - what happened on 9-11 with the cell phones? People said, "I love you." When the planes were crashing, it was "I love you." What did you say when you left home this morning? "Don't forget to pick up the laundry?" In our family, everybody says I love you all the time. I don't think they even know they're saying it. Kids call you on the phone. "Okay dad, love you." It's a wonderful reflex. I walk out of the house; my wife is always saying, "drive carefully." It drives me nuts. How many years can I hear her tell me to drive carefully? But she loves me, so she's always noticing even a little bit of dust on your clothing if you're going out. She's saying, "Let me fix you up." And that's out of love.

One other thing we can learn from is criticism. This is important for the medical profession as well as others. The Sufi poet Rumi said, "Criticism polishes your mirror." In those days, mirrors were metal. You polished and you saw more. But when I read that, I thought, "That's a wonderful message." If you want to find a good doctor, find one who gets criticized by patients, family and nurses. How do you know they're good? Because they're listening to the criticism. If you never accept criticism, people will stop criticizing you because they know you're always making excuses. You say, "That's not my fault, you're a terrible patient, okay, goodbye." Take it as a positive sign if you get feedback or criticism, listen and learn from it. I think that's the most important.

The other couple of quotes that say a lot to me include one from the book by William Saroyan, The Human Comedy. In the book, a young man dies in the war, very similar to what's going on right now if your brother died in Iraq. And his friend says to him, "The best part of a good man stays forever, for love is immortal and makes all things immortal, but hate dies every minute." And the other was Thornton Wilder's The Bridge of San Luis Ray. There's a passage where this bridge breaks and three or four people are killed. The priest is looking for what they did right and what they did wrong as they were on the bridge, but he ultimately realizes this is not about any of that. The last paragraph in the book says, "And we ourselves shall be loved for a while and forgotten, but the love will have been enough." All those impulses of love return to the love that made them, even memory is not necessary for love. There's the land of the living and the land of the dead and the bridge is love, the only survival, the only meaning.

The other thing - to get mystical for a minute or two. When you talk, especially to parents of children who have died, you hear stories about the kids coming back, as crazy as this may sound. I've had, again, not being a normal doctor, I've had mystics come to me and tell me of my patients who have died and what they had to tell me. And they brought exact quotes. Number one, they'd come in and say the person's name - Frank, Randy. These are people in the support group telling me this, and others are my patients. They say, "This is what someone says they wanted you to know." They would use the deceased person's expressions and their terms. I truly believe, as I said, that our bodies die. But, our consciousness goes on. My latest meditation, in a sense that helped me understand this, is: "We're like water. Consciousness is like water. When you watch a stream, the water bounces off rocks, can get over dams, can get through all kinds of troubles, goes back to where it started. It can turn into vapor and come back again as water. That part of us recycles too, consciousness." If we move up in the scale - for example, if you become a college student and your level of consciousness rises, then you're helping the future. Because those who come after you, will have some of that awareness. If you are a destructive individual who remains in first grade, so to speak, then life is going to be a lot harder after you. You're not advancing the course of creation.

When we come close to death, we're all going to say, "Forget the borders, forget the races, forget the religions. We've got to become a family." As a surgeon, that's what I learned. We're all the same color inside. The differences are for recognition, but inside, we're all the same.

http://berniesiegelmd.com/

Dr. Ian Gawler

Cancer Survivor
The Gawler Foundation, Australia

Back in 1975, I was a young veterinarian. I was also a decathlon athlete. I had some time off. I had been playing football through the winter. I got back into my athletic training. Then, I found I had soreness in my right thigh that fairly rapidly started to swell and turned out to be an osteogenic sarcoma, which is a fairly virulent form of bone cancer. At the time, the treatment recommended was to have my leg amputated through the hip, which was done early in 1975. I was given the impression I had about a five percent chance of being alive in five year's time. As it turned out, the cancer reoccurred in less than a year. At that stage, I'd been in the medical libraries and I couldn't find a record of anyone who'd lived more than six months with that sort of diagnosis. It was pretty clear that in those days there was very little that conventional medicine could do to extend my life.

That thought didn't appeal to me very much. I was pretty keen on life itself. I think I was fortunate in a couple of ways. I think firstly, as a veterinarian, I'd been quite used to seeing animals heal in a whole range of conditions. I had grown to have quite a respect for this innate healing potential that animals have. I thought that perhaps there might be a way of stimulating a similar sort of healing from within my own body, given the right circumstances.

I think, also, it's helpful to observe how the mind works. If I'd stayed with my scientific training and accepted the evidence out of the literature of the time, which was that nobody survived this situation longer than six months - if I'd accepted that, then I don't think it would have been at all difficult to have been punctual and die on time. It raises that whole question of hope. I think, for myself, I was almost foolhardy enough to go against the evidence of the day and to hope that it was possible to survive. As such though, I thought, "Well, it's probably not going to happen just by accident, just by good luck." I think there's a huge difference between what you can call wishful thinking - which is where you hope for the best and don't do anything about it - and what I would consider authentic, positive thinking to be, which is where you hope for the best and you actually do a lot about it.

I guess with that thought I felt that it may be quite possible to recover. And that perhaps the means was through activating this internal potential for healing that the body has. I thought, "Well, how are you going to do that?" I was fortunate. Having been trained as a veterinarian, we had a lot of training in nutrition. When it was put to me that nutrition might actually help the body to heal in a difficult situation like cancer, I thought, "Well yeah, that's a possibility." So I got very enthused about that and looked into it in great detail. I found a lot of benefit in it.

But then, also, I had a sort of latent interest in the spiritual path and meditation. I was very fortunate to be around in those pioneering days of mind/body medicine. I was doubly fortunate that one of the great pioneers of meditation as a therapy, Dr. Ainslie Meares, was actually living and working in Melbourne, Australia which was my hometown at the time. Dr. Meares had come out of a background of hypnotherapy. Through his particular interest in pain management, he had discovered meditation back in the 60s - well before it was being used anywhere else in a real therapeutic setting. He was very extraordinary, I think, in terms of his capacity to recognize the potential that meditation had - not only for helping people to manage pain, but to bring the body back into its natural balance. This would facilitate healing across a wide range of physical and psychological conditions.

He had been very much involved in that as the focus of his medical practice for many years. He finally went public and posited this idea that meditation might actually help people. That was just the time I was diagnosed with secondary. So, I sort of teamed forces with him, learned the style of meditation that he recommended, which is a stillness-based form of meditation. I practiced that very intensively. The state of mind that developed out of that, sort of built on what was a fairly naturally positive state of mind, which I had to begin with. Looking at a whole range of complementary and alternative medicines, I was also considering what could be done for me medically, eventually putting this whole sort of package together.

I surprised everybody, including myself somewhat, and got well. Then it got really interesting because this was the middle of '78, when I was well. I went back to my original doctors and the majority of them reacted in a quite unexpected way. I thought they'd be actually quite pleased and interested in what had happened. Unfortunately, they actually reacted by getting angry with me. It was almost like I got well for the wrong reasons. They didn't like the thought that diet might be therapeutic or meditation might be therapeutic. These were quite radical ideas back in the 70s. So I had to adjust to that. It really surprised me as a veterinarian. I thought it was a very peculiar response.

As the years went on, I went back into my veterinary practice. I increasingly got letters - or had people actually come into my veterinary practice. They'd heard that I'd recovered against the odds in an unusual way and were inquiring as to whether anything I'd done might be helpful for them. So this idea of starting a self-help based cancer support group had its genesis right in my own personal experience and in the volume of people that inquired. Ainslie Meares had written up my story in the Medical Journal of Australia as a case report, in 1978. That had led to the media getting hold of it, and it sort of became fairly widely known. But it wasn't until 1981, that I started running these groups. Really from the start we had this dual intention of helping people very much with their quality of life and the experience that having cancer led to for them. We wanted to help them find meaning and purpose through that, but also our focus was how they could actually help extend their lives and hopefully recover.

So, from those rather tentative beginnings back in the early 80s, that intention flourished into the Foundation I work for now, which has about fifty members on staff. We run residential programs for people with cancer. We've also expanded into running programs, lifestyle-based self-help programs, for people with MS, which are going very well. But also, we realized that these principles we were using to help people get well had very much to do with living well. It really is very much a lifestyle-based program.

So, for people who don't have illness and are basically well to start with, these same principles are terrific for preventing illness and for actually being really well. That's sort of taken us in the domain of wellness programs and lifestyle-based programs. That brings us up to where we are now.

If we address the question of hope, I think it's really important. In the clinical experience I've had over all these years now, I think it's useful to identify five actual distinct levels of hope - with the first one being hopelessness or lack of hope. Anybody who's been in a situation where they feel hopeless knows what a black sort of place that is to be in.

I think often when people are first diagnosed with a life-threatening illness, that's what they feel, particularly if bad news is given to them badly. I think it's a real challenge for the medical profession to address this issue. I think still too many people are being given bad news badly, in a way that takes hope away. That leads to despair, despondency, and actually a whole raft of unpleasant outcomes.

I think when people have moved through that first stage, the next stage - or the second stage of hope - is actually hope to survive. So often when people talk of the will to live, in fact, I think they can be talking of the will not to die. It's actually more about avoiding dying than actually getting well. As such, there's often a lot of fear in that sort of level of hope. People often become quite vulnerable; they often fluctuate in their emotional and mental states quite rapidly. Like when things seem to be going well, they're up. If they get a setback of some sort, they tend to crash pretty badly. They tend to clutch at straws. They can have an air of desperation, an air of panic about them in that stage of hope.

The third stage of hope is where there's hope for a better future. I think it's where a lot of people function in their daily lives. It's sort of like, well, whatever is going on at the moment, it's not too bad - but it's not terrific. And, if I do something about it in the future, it's going to get better. So there's a sense of having some control, having some sense of order and being able to plan to do something about the conditions that you're in. But the underlying issue is that, at the moment, there's dissatisfaction. There's an underlying tension or anxiety and a wish for things to get better in the future, along with the thought that real happiness is in the future rather than where I am at the moment. I think a lot of people function in that level of hope through a lot of their lives.

Often in the fourth level is where you're differentiating, because it's similar, but the significant difference is the hope for a spiritual realization. So, it might be that people come to terms with their physical, material wealth or circumstances, the state of their relationships, their mind, and things like that. But there's still a sense of something lacking, there's something more to life, and I haven't actually got it. That is a real sense of spiritual connectedness. So again, that may lead to the spiritual path or going back to church or whatever it is. There's some sense I can do something about that. Again, somewhere off in the future, I can have this spiritual realization and things will be better.

Then the fifth stage of hope is where the hope is actually for the present moment. There's a sort of realization that fantasizing about things getting better in the future is all well and good. Planning for it and doing something about it may be better, but it would be even better, again, if you could be content and happy in the present moment. So, how we can break free of traumas or difficulties - or longing for the past and any hopes, and perhaps even fears, for the future - and find peace of mind and contentedness in the present moment? That's one of the things we really try and help people with when they come to our programs. How can you find this enduring peace of mind that's independent of the past or the future, independent of your external circumstances and has much more to do with this inner state of mind?

I think if you look at the way many people are diagnosed with cancer, it's easy to see there are some real difficulties in the way it's handled culturally. I mention that quite often. I think bad news is given badly in the sense that many doctors, I think, have the view that their job is to be open and honest. But they get confused between the difference between statistics and individuals. So, they talk to an individual in statistical terms. If the statistics for a given cancer are good, stating a ninety percent chance of a five-year survival, doctors tend to be quite positive in a way that'll sort of present the diagnosis and the treatment. I often hear people who have been diagnosed with Hodgkin's disease say they are being told they were lucky. I haven't met anyone who felt lucky, because as an individual, you've still got a crappy situation to deal with. As time goes on, that crappy situation may transform into something meaningful and purposeful. But at the time, it doesn't feel like much of a blessing - unless these people who are diagnosed have got a fairly enlightened state of mind to begin with.

But for the majority, what happens if they're in a situation where the five-year survival is difficult? Or, particularly, what if they get a recurrence where the odds can significantly be decreased for long-term survival? Then, if that's expressed in statistical terms, it often can be quite damning in terms of how to fix the sense of that person's hope. Compound that with the fact that the way a lot of medical treatment is carried out. It tends to be quite disempowering. So, people who are used to being in control of their life situation, perhaps their work, their family, things like that, are suddenly thrust into an environment in which they don't have a lot of familiarity - like the medical system. It's clearly quite a technical and sort of an alien environment to a lot of people when they first come into it. It's clear that there's a lot of fear around cancer, both in terms of the actual diagnosis and treatment. The reality is that a lot of treatments for cancer are tough. Nobody likes having bits of them removed or going through chemotherapy and radiotherapy. Even when they work well, they're still often really tough on people. So, there's a lot to be fearful of. There's a lot of natural anxiety.

There's also this dilemma for a lot of people in terms of the decisions we have to make - and have to be made quickly. The problem with that is this: If somebody has been given a diagnosis that causes a lot of fear, it's very easy for them to panic and to be in a really confused state of mind. This is actually a terrible state of mind in which to be making important decisions. The reality is that in most cancer situations, unless there's actually a medical emergency - which means you're calling an ambulance or getting to an emergency room - there are very few decisions whereby waiting for a week or two will actually affect the long-term outcome.

I would suggest, for most people, that following a diagnosis of cancer, it's a really intelligent choice just to think, "I'm going to take a week or two to stand back from this. I'll allow myself to get over the initial impact and the emotional affect, the mental effect of the diagnosis, and try and integrate that with my family and friends somewhat. I'll let my mind clear a little and then go back and actually address what are we actually going to do about this - and consider that in a measured way."

The other thing that I think is important is that cancer is essentially a lifestyle illness. We know that the major things that are identified in the medical mainstream that cause cancer are lifestyle issues - like what you eat, whether you smoke or not, what sort of things you drink. Then, there are all sorts of things like the environmental factors. It's largely a lifestyle illness, very much like heart disease or Type II diabetes. Anybody who is diagnosed with either of those conditions today, their doctors are almost negligent if they don't talk to them about their lifestyle in the first consultation. I think the same situation exists in cancer meds. I think the fact that lifestyle isn't addressed early in the illness is a real oversight. From the individual's point of view, it's actually an area of neglect. Because, in my view, anyone who's diagnosed with cancer - just as with heart disease or type II diabetes - should be encouraged to consider what's going on in their lifestyle from the point of that first diagnosis. The reason for that is that it's likely their lifestyle has something to do with the cause of their condition. So, getting rid of causes, changing things that you're doing that are provoking the cancer, makes sense.

Whatever treatment people go through, a healthy lifestyle is going to support them to both endure the treatment and to get the best out of it. Then there's this real prospect that's showing up very strongly in modern research that a healthy lifestyle actually has therapeutic value in its own right. So, I think if you look at the current research, it's very reasonable to say that if you compare somebody with an unhealthy lifestyle who gets diagnosed with cancer with somebody with a healthy lifestyle, the person with the healthy lifestyle is likely to live twice as long as the person who has a really crappy lifestyle.

It's a very strange thing that goes on. Those with Type II diabetes think the general community understands that this relates to lifestyle. The scientific evidence for it is really strong. But with cancer medicine, it's almost like there's a blind spot to it. There's not nearly the interest in researching that area. In fact, a bit like the way my doctors responded when I recovered, some medical people are actually quite antagonistic about even considering the option.

It's hard, I think, to really understand it. It seems like there's almost an over-concern about relating people's lifestyle to their health, when it comes to cancer. I think it's just confusion. When you do actually look into your past with the right state of mind - which is not with a sense of recrimination through shame or guilt or blame - but you look back and see the connection between what you were doing in the past and what's going on now, in terms of your health, you'll realize that these things are linked. Then you realize you can actually change your lifestyle. It's very empowering. You can change the whole dynamic of the illness. Instead of living a lifestyle that's led to an illness forming, you can actually turn the tables around and create a regenerative, healing lifestyle.

If we consider how meditation can actually help with healing, I think it's worth talking about four areas. The first one is that meditation actually helps us to make good and healthy decisions. When it comes to our health, it's clearly our mind that's the major factor.

It's our mind that decides what we eat. It's our mind that decides whether we exercise and what we drink, what sort of treatments we have. The mind is the key factor.

To make good decisions, we need a couple things. We need good information and we need the clarity of mind to sort out the choices that are available. We need to make good effective choices for us personally. That's where meditation is a real strength, because it leads to that clarity of mind. It helps us to deal with the conflicting issues of old habits and beliefs and emotions that can actually muddle our thinking. So, the first thing that meditation does is lead to clear thinking and good decision-making.

The second thing is that when we meditate, particularly in the way I would suggest that's good for our health, we learn how to relax physically in quite a deep way. At the same time, we calm our minds. As such, we enter into a great state that's attuned to a deep, physiological rest. The consequence of that is that our body comes back to this natural balance; our physiology comes back into a natural balance. Then the underlying principle is that when the body's in its natural state of balance, it's exquisitely well designed to both prevent illness and to be healthy, to heal. I think that the normal state for the body is a healthy state. You have to acquire an illness. You acquire an illness when things get out of balance. Meditation restores that natural balance.

Even more, though, not only does meditation restore the balance in the physical sense, but also it brings emotional balance. People find it easy to be authentic in their emotional life. It leads to this clarity of mind that we've already spoken about. People find it easier to make good decisions and to commit to following them through - so things tend to get done better.

Also, there's a balance in the spiritual life that comes. There's a sense of connectedness that gives people a real deep confidence. That's the second and most direct way in which meditation helps us achieve this natural state of balance.

The third area is imagery, which is the more active use of the mind. This is where we can use the active mind to actually stimulate healing through learning about mind/body medicine and using it in that more active way.

The fourth way that our meditation can impact on our health is through our state of mind. Again, this is a bit like the first one. But it's more to do with the fact that when we meditate, our state of mind tends to just naturally gravitate toward the life-affirming and healing-type qualities. So, when you meditate there's a natural optimism that comes out. There's a natural positivity where we find it easier to be joyful and to laugh at things. So our state of mind improves. Our state of mind is directly related to our health, of course. Meditation in that sense can be a very good and direct antidote for depression, a very reliable way of helping treat anxiety, and a very reliable way of generating a sustainable level of well-being.

A way of conceptualizing this is that the balance that we're talking of is a bit like a spinning top. If you've got a top that's spinning, it stays in balance. You can give it a little nudge and it'll wobble a bit and then it comes back into balance. If you give it a real whack, you can knock it right off balance, and you've got to really do something major to start it up again.

The body is actually designed to be healthy. Its natural

state is to be healthy. If we were to think of a good definition for health, I think it's "a dynamic state of balance." The body, fortunately, is designed for the fact that life goes up and down, physically. Our environment changes, and from time to time, we might knock ourselves around or have some illness to deal with. Emotionally, most people's lives go up and down. Mine certainly does. Mentally, our state can vary. But there's this clear and powerful principle in medicine called homeostasis, which is the fact that the body is actually designed to keep coming back into balance all the time. It's got an incredible raft of mechanisms, both physical and psychological, to help us to do that. Clearly, in day-to-day life, the balance that we'd ideally like to be in, gets rattled a bit.

What meditation can do is help to give us a time, where in a formal sense each day, we actually let go of the busyness of the day. We let go of the physical activity; we let go of the thoughts that we're engaged in. We let everything go into this state of deep physiological rest and return to that natural state of balance. The curious thing, and the wonderful thing about that, is that if you do that even ten or twenty minutes once or twice a day, that sense of balance becomes increasingly pervading through the day and it stays with you. So that stability, that balance, becomes more durable and reliable. It's well demonstrated that people who meditate regularly have much less illness in their lives. If we're thinking about how we can restore our health, how we can practice healing, then meditation is one of the premier ways in which you can help the body to actually bring about healing from within.

The other good thing about it is that it's very complementary in synergistic terms with other forms of treatment. There's nothing about meditation that conflicts with medical treatment. In fact, it's likely to reinforce it very strongly. It certainly reinforces counseling or psychotherapy. It's lovely to be an advocate for meditation because it's so easy. It's got so many benefits.

I think when it comes to life, there are some basic questions we have to sort out if we want to live a conscious and aware life. One of them is: Do things happen for a reason or just by accident? If there's a rhyme and a reason running through life - which is a much more appealing thought and certainly the one that I would operate from - then it's almost like going through a school situation where lessons come along. You get a chance to learn things, and then you get tested. So often the things that we find challenging in our life are like these tests. They're an opportunity for us to find out what we've learned, how well we can apply what we've learned. As such, if there's actually some order in life, it wouldn't make sense to give tests that were beyond someone's capacity. If you were running a school, it wouldn't make sense to give your kindergarten kids the university exam. It would just be nonsense.

I think as a general principle, whenever somebody is faced with a challenge, I strongly support the view that they've got the potential to meet it. Sometimes these challenges can bring out resources or capacities in people that they may not have been so aware of. But, I think it's a truth that it's often in the difficult times of life that we learn what's most important. Often when life is treating us easily, kindly - life is just rolling along - we can tend to take it for granted. It's very easy for the years to go by and then you suddenly look back and think, "What the heck was that all about?" Many people, and certainly people I work with, and the great majority, find that when they're faced with these really difficult life circumstances, it really causes them to consider their priorities and their choices - what's really important to them. As such, they very often come to the conclusion that despite the difficulties, the major traumas, the difficulties in this sense, the challenges are actually worthwhile and certainly meaningful.

I would rather have worked all this stuff out without having to go through the illness and having my leg amputated and all that stuff. But given that's not what happened, and given that I did go through those difficulties, it's easy to look back and see the benefit of it in my own life.

I think if you're thinking about your health, your capacity for healing and your well-being, and that's like a relatively new thought - up to that point you've just been living your life - suddenly, you realize that actually you can take more control over this. I think the first thing to realize is the importance of the mind. When we consider the mind's role in this, there are two things that are wonderful about it. The first one is that we can change it. We often laugh and think that changing the mind is a woman's prerogative. The good news is that everybody can do it. The mind is incredibly flexible, actually, if we realize that. The second thing is that you can actually train your mind. So when you start to connect the dots, if you get a sense that what you're doing in your life isn't working so well - or the circumstances of your life don't suit you, either because of physical illness or state of relationships or the state of your mind - then I think that the next important thing is to recognize the power of hope and to recognize that you can do something about it. If the hope, to start with, is just that you can get some relief from the suffering you're in, that's very real. There's a reliable way out of suffering if you use your mind intelligently.

Then it's a matter of, I think, applying the two key principles in this area. That is the value of learning and practicing. So really to get the benefit out of what we're talking about you have to learn about it. You actually have to study it. Then you have to put it into practice. It's a bit like two wings of a bird. A bird needs two wings to fly. Without either of those wings of study and practice, I think it's very difficult, actually. I guess that points to the need to find good instruction - like what books you can read, what are the groups you can go to, who the people are that can help you learn about this area. And then, how do you take a theory and actually put it into practice, so that you can embody it and it actually becomes real in your life?

I think it's helpful to encourage people. I see a lot of people who come to groups, who I meet along the way, who are really struggling with difficult circumstances. They've had this sort of glimmer of hope and have recognized that they can do something about their circumstances. They've really worked on it to great effect. Ideally they'll get to this point where, again - rather than hoping for something off in the future - they actually get to a point where they can find this happiness in their present moment and be really content day by day.

I think that's where people get into - yes, karma is a good word for it - a certain mindset, but with probably a more secular, Western view. You can talk more about the power of belief and habit, but where does that come from - the power of belief? I think from current life experience and perhaps a hangover from previous karma as well. Yeah,

I think it can be difficult sometimes, frustrating.

It's very frustrating when you know what's good for somebody else and they won't do it. It's something I've had to learn. For this stuff to be useful, it's got to actually come from individual concern. I think in a situation like I'm in, that's part of the deal. You ask how do I find a way to inspire people and motivate people? How can I help them to realize what's possible and to break free of unhealthy habits or conditioning?

People come here in a whole range of situations. In the early days it was more as a last resort. But I think more and more people are realizing the importance of, if they're dealing with illness, dealing with this early in the illness and making it a part of the strategy they have for managing the illness.

I guess there are an increasing number of people who are basically well and waking up and thinking about what sort of old age they want to have. They ask what sort of health they want to have day by day. And again, they are appreciating the fact that they can do something about it. We get the whole range of people.

The healthy programs are lovely to run. In a way, people have said I did something significant in recovering from the illness. Really, that's just sort of self-preservation kicking in. I don't think there's anything all that honorable about it in that sense. I might have had the determination to carry it through, but the people I really admire are the people who are well and who take account of the preciousness of their life. They actually want to do something with it while they're well. I was, in a sense, sort of forced into all this from my circumstances. I meet people who are well and used to waking up to the fact that this life is so precious.

They realize they can do something really useful with it and want to get the best out of it. That's very commendable.

http://www.iangawler.com/

Susan Ryan Jordan

Breast Cancer Survivor
Author

I was diagnosed with breast cancer in 1979, October of 1979, and it's funny because I always remember being afraid of getting breast cancer - that it was one of my great fears. I had just been divorced from my former husband, my mother had just died, I was separated from my children for a brief period, and I thought that basically my life was over. This was before I was even diagnosed.

I thought that would be the worst possible thing that could ever happen to a woman - to have cancer. When I was diagnosed with it, basically people thought of it as a death sentence. You did not pick up the newspaper and read as you do today, that cancer can be thought of as a chronic illness. Cancer in those days was something people didn't even talk about. You never even said the word "breast." You didn't say "cancer." I mean, it was one of those things that was very quiet and never discussed.

But for some reason I was fearful that I, myself, would get it. Then came a feeling that I deserved it. This was because I had, in my mind, back then, failed as a woman. I'd failed in those roles that are supposed to be, again, a cultural thing - in those roles that people always impressed upon women - be a good wife, be a good mother, be a good daughter. I felt I failed in all three of those areas, so a diagnosis of breast cancer would be the perfect punishment. Talk about a messed-up psyche. That's what I had back in those days.

The diagnosis was that I had an aggressive form of breast cancer. In those days they did not tell you Stage One, Stage Two, Stage Three. My biopsy was done at a surgeon's office in New Haven, Connecticut. The surgeon was a member of the Yale faculty. He was the best one that I had heard of and I went to see him. I was teaching at a private school and this group was in their health plan so I went to see him, happily. It turned out to be for the absolute best, as it all turned out.

He performed a biopsy. My husband now, Pat, was with me in the waiting room while we waited. I'll never forget. The doctor came rushing in and looked absolutely shocked. He had gotten the results immediately. He brought us back to his office. I sat down. I fully expected this, so I was not really shocked. He said, "You have breast cancer. It's aggressive. But the lump is small - so let's just take it from there, schedule the operation and go in and have this modified radical mastectomy." That is what happened on that particular October day, back in 1979.

My surgeon was William McCullough. His partner was Bernie Siegel. There was another doctor there, Richard Seltzer, who had just retired, having written what turned out to be a best-seller of his own called Mortal Lessons, I think was the name. Bernie had just met a wonderful doctor, an oncologist, named Carl Simonton.

On the day that I was diagnosed, I left the office with a book that Bernie's nurse handed to me and said, "Go home and read this." The name of the book was Getting Well Again by Carl Simonton. And I remember taking the book, getting in my car, putting it on the seat of the car and thinking, "nobody gets well again from cancer, but I'll read it anyway."

So I went back to school. I was teaching at Rosemary Hall, and after I did all my house mother duties and finished all my lesson plans, I was just seized with this panic. I thought, "I don't really know what I'm going to do here." I had visions of myself dead - what will happen to my children - and I remember thinking, "I just do not want to die. I can't." I had just met Pat. I thought "I can't, I can't, I can't possibly die." I grabbed the book and I read it, and I read it one night. And it had a profound influence. Basically it was a challenge to patients who had just been diagnosed with cancer to heal themselves. It was a book that explained that it was possible. It was so full of hope, that I took every single solitary word of that and I applied it to my own life.

The Doctor, Simonton, and his then wife, who was a psychologist who worked with people who were unusual achievers - people who had an unordinary drive to do well and succeed - had made a study, I think I'm right, of a hundred cancer patients. Those that had this extraordinary will to succeed survived long after they were supposed to have died. They kept coming back for their annual checkups - ten, twenty years later. So, she and he wondered if those personality traits could be taught to people who had been diagnosed with cancer, and if they can be taught, what the results would be. And I thought, "Well, if other people did it, then I will. And I will do it."

They mentioned something like setting goals, small ones. Don't bite off more than you can chew in one day, but set yourself very small goals - minute to minute even. Get through the lesson plan; teach the one class; finish the day; then look forward to tomorrow. Little by little by little, and tell yourself that you can. And then they encouraged you to be very much in tune with what your own body can do for you, and to use your imagination regarding how you're going to make yourself well. Don't be afraid to just use your imagination.

In the beginning I did set those very small goals for myself. I can remember setting them. Get up in the morning, make the coffee. Okay, that's done. Now pick up the lesson plan. This is going to be class one, grammar. Class two, Jane Eyre. Class three, history of theatrical arts.

Then I thought to myself, "Well, they said to imagine your body. There are parts of it that you can't see that you're never going to see. You're not this CAT scan thing that you can look inside and say, 'Look. Everything is going this way and that way.'" They said imagine the cancer, so I did imagine it as this black type of octopus that I hated, and then I imagined my immune system as this little army of white soldiers.

I had read in this book that the immune system cannot tolerate cancer cells because they're weak and confused, so I said, "Go for it." I would imagine the soldiers rushing to where this cancer was and beating up on it, literally destroying them, having a battle royal in there. To this day, I can still do it. Your whole body feels as though it's charged. Literally, you get pins and needles. I can literally do this any time I want. Your imagination is quite a powerful thing when it comes to how your body responds to it. Basically, it's your mind informing your body, which is what it's supposed to do to start with.

So I envisioned this. Then I said, "What's happening to all these dead cancer cells? I'm not having them floating around in there." So, I would get up and drink water, and then everything would kind of flush out. And I thought,

"Great, I'm getting rid of this little by little by little."

Then I went into the hospital and had the mastectomy.

When I went in, I went through a CAT scan. I remember saying to myself, "Don't think funny thoughts in this tube." It was very scary. If you're at all claustrophobic, you're lying in there and you're thinking, "Ugh, what is it seeing that I can't see?" I remember saying to myself, "Don't think these crazy thoughts because your body will then react in a crazy fashion. Be totally calm." So I was.

I was wheeled back upstairs and waited and waited and waited. I thought that an anesthesiologist was supposed to come in and see me about the next morning, when the operation was supposed to take place. But he didn't come. I guess about eight or nine o'clock at night I began to wonder what is the matter here? A technician came up again and said, "They would like another CAT scan because they think that something is wrong somehow with your liver." I didn't have any idea. The idea that cancer could have spread to my liver, I'd never even thought of. I just thought, "All right, I'll go and do the CAT scan. I'll get it over with. I would like to go to sleep, get up in the morning, get the thing done and get the heck out of here." That was my view. Perfectly healthy view, when I look back now. Exactly the way I should have been thinking.

The second CAT scan came back fine. I woke up the next morning, had this mastectomy, and basically, I always thought that was the start of my new life.

After the mastectomy I had a few complications. I hemorrhaged almost. A friend of mine who was a resident there said to me, "You almost bought the ranch on that one." But I'm sitting here. I survived that. Tests were very long in coming back. It was a little nerve-wracking. I spent ten days in the hospital basically recovering and waiting, waiting for these tests. Each day that I spent in that hospital, I spent doing those same visualizations.

Finally, on the day that I went home, my surgeon, Dr. Bill McCullough, came in and he said, "I'm really surprised. But I'm very happy to tell you that there's no cancer anywhere." He said, "You don't have it. We were very, very worried about you. But it's gone."

I never questioned it. I said, "Good. I'm out of here."

Whenever somebody is given an idea that they are mortal after all, I'm sure those people would think the way I do. When you're faced with your own mortality, you realize your life is to be lived in the way that you decide you're going to live. For me, this meant that I was going to pursue the things that make me happy. That I was no longer going to worry about what people thought, that I was no longer going to worry about being the perfect, perfect person. Perfect mother, the perfect daughter, the perfect wife. I felt it was very important to live fully, to appreciate everything around me. To be in charge of my own destiny, and by all means, to reconnect with who I really was - and I'd lost sight of that. I think a lot of women do when they're raised the way I was, in particular.

And I found that true with the many, many breast cancer patients that I've talked to over the years. They're always so busy trying to please everybody else. If you ask them, "Who's the most important person in your life?" They don't say, "Well I am." They've lost sight of the self that they truly are. So busy trying to live up to other people's expectations of themselves. So that's what I came away with. I wanted to find out who I really was. I made a promise to myself that I was not ever going to deny that.

Dis-ease is such a great name for illness because it means that you are not at ease. You are not at ease with yourself. I know for me, I'm convinced that it was the sense of having failed, in my mind's eye, having failed other people. No sense whatsoever of the value that I had to myself as a person. It was that sense of loss, which I think is a tremendous component of dis-ease, a sense of grief, a sense of guilt. All of those things weigh very, very heavily on the mind. They weigh very heavily on the spirit.

Go back to Shakespeare. I'll never forget reading *Macbeth* years later, years after I was diagnosed. When Lady Macbeth is afflicted, her husband says to the physician, "Can't you route that out of her? Can't you get that uneasiness away, that guilt out of her?" And the physician says, "No. Therein the patient must take care of herself."

So you have to go back deep into yourself and understand what it was that made you so uneasy, so filled with unease, so filled with guilt, so filled with loss, so filled with despair, which is just a giving up. Then you must take every precaution never to let yourself feel those thoughts again, because they hurt. I know that's what happened to me. I know that having realized that, that realization made me well.

I would not wish to ever have it again, certainly. But having had it and looking back, I think that I learned things that I never would have learned otherwise, without any doubt.

My own particular view about why there is such a prevalence of cancer these days, and this is my view; I don't think people are careful enough about taking care of themselves. I mean people will say, "I don't eat fat, or I go and have a blood test every year and I'm always careful about my cholesterol," but that is taking care of your physical self. That is not taking care of the spiritual you.

If you go back and think about the time you were the happiest as a kid, the time you felt the most free, if you can remember that - that's the self that you were. And that's the self that you should never lose. But I think people do that. I think it isn't just breast cancer, it's, say, prostate cancer. Many, many times you'll hear that a man has come down with prostate cancer after he has just been fired from his job. Maybe six months to a year, year-and-a-half later. It's that sense of living for something else, rather than living within. I think people tend to try to please, and I think that they feel failure. And many of these people can't express that failure or express that loss or express that guilt. What are other people going to think? Maybe as a culture we're too worried about that.

There are stresses associated with it, with cancer. No doubt about it in my mind. I have always felt, ever since my own experience with cancer, that when you're sitting in that hospital bed or the doctor's office and you receive a diagnosis of cancer, not only should the surgeon be sitting there, but a good psychiatrist should be sitting there too. A wonderful therapist should be sitting there. Perhaps a trusted friend should be sitting there. The issue is not simply physical. It just is not.

There is a wonderful foundation in California called the Heal Breast Cancer Foundation. I was happy to go out there where I received an award for my book, The Immune Spirit. I was so happy to be able to be part of that because these people are saying that the causes of cancer are not simply something that you pick up from breathing something nasty in the air - or that you're trying to be the best possible person at your job. They are saying that there is literally an association between cancer and what happens with your immune system when you suffer a loss, when you suffer a separation, when you feel despair. It's an absolute letting go of all your inner resources - that's what leads to an illness like that. And that's why you've got to be so vigilant about taking care of the "you."

It's not a question of "don't eat certain foods," it's a question of saying, "Hey wait a minute, I don't like that you're doing that, or this is really what I believe - listen to me. I'm important." It's that sense of confidence of self, and that sense of strength of spirit, that when you lose that, I think you're absolutely prone to cancer, and that's my own view - having lived through that kind of thing.

I think people do need to take responsibility for their health. I would like to put it in that way, which is a very positive way. Many physicians will say to you, "Oh gee whiz, I don't want to make you feel guilty because you got sick." But people are responsible for their inner health, of course they are.

Here's something else that I'd like to bring out. People look at things in different ways. When you talk about stressful situations, what is stressful for person A might not be stressful for person B. Take for example, sitting and waiting in an airport. Here you have person A, who absolutely loves to fly, can't wait to get on the airplane. "I want to look down and see the world from above." Here's person B who thinks, "I hate this. I can't stand it." Person A never gets sweaty palms. Person B is a nervous wreck. It's the same airplane. It's the same airport. It's the same flight. But it's the different way that the flight is looked at. We don't see things as they are; we see things as we are. So it involves tremendous self-introspection, self-discovery, to ask yourself, "How come I look at this in such a way that it's making me nervous? Why do I do that?"

That's what I wrote about. It occurred to me, while I was getting well that I looked at things in ways that were not healthy. I looked at things in fearful ways. I looked at things the way my mother used to. "Oh my God, what will happen now? What will people think? You never know what's going to happen. You've got to always be careful. You've got to be prepared." Rather than say, "Don't worry about it." The difference I was writing about, between my mother and my grandmother - my grandmother never gave - as she would say - a hoot. She was a very strong, self-aware person within. My mother was not. I picked up the lessons from my mother. I started looking at things in fearful ways. One of the things that I realized in my recovery was that, in order to stay well, I better start looking at the world the way my grandmother used to. It was that kind of process of self-discovery.

The way you look at things is what you inherit. You do not inherit the genetic makeup for cancer, I don't think. You inherit the lessons that you learned as a kid, as a kid growing up. My grandmother used to say, "I don't care what people think." My mother would say, "But you have to worry. My God. Wear this hat. Don't wear the beret to church that your Aunt Lucille brought you back from Paris, France because if you did wear that in Fairfield, Connecticut, people would think you were a bohemian." My grandmother said, "That hat looks so smart. I would wear that every Sunday." So there's the difference. Thank God I had her in my life. But I grew up much more under the influence of my mother. I grew up as a Catholic -

always told to be a good girl. The good girl is the unselfish girl. Think of everybody else first.

So it's no wonder that you grow up with this set of ideas that you've inherited, that you see all around you. It's tremendously important. It is what you inherit from your behavior, the way that you perceive the world is what you get, and then your body follows suit.

If I were to meet someone who is just diagnosed with breast cancer, I would say to them, first of all, the most comforting thing I could think of: "This is a glitch, it's a bump in the road. You'll be fine. This is something that you will get rid of and never have again." That would be the very first thing I would say because that is comfort, and that is what you want to give, and you want to give hope. Then I would say, "What's been going on in your life, especially in the last eighteen months? Has there been a loss?" If I were able to speak very freely to this person: has there been a loss, has there been a disappointment, have you felt grief, have you lost hope? Why? Let's think about those things.

Then, once that response came back I would say, "Can you even imagine the number of women who have had the same thing happen?" There is safety in numbers. Patients feel a tremendous amount of comfort of not only seeing somebody who survived breast cancer 28 years ago or 30 years ago or 35 years ago - there's tremendous hope in knowing that - but there's also tremendous hope in knowing that so many people have felt the same and that this has happened to people that felt that way and they got over it. That would be the second thing I would say.

I would say that along with the doctor, and what he has prescribed for you, think of this as a journey of self-discovery. Go back into your past. I would tell them to do what I did. Go back and ask, "How come I thought of things the way I did?" Let me think of all those lessons that I learned when I was a child. Why did I think that because this happened, it only happened to me? Why did I think that because this happened, I failed? Why did I think the negative things? Why didn't I think the positive, happy things?

I would strongly suggest that along with the physical help that the doctors are giving you, do some real interesting self-discovery digging. It's a heck of a journey.

By all means, I would encourage those kinds of visualizations. Imagination is a remarkable tool to make yourself well. The more vivid the imagination the better, and you can make your imagination more and more vivid, you can have a whole lot of fun doing that. Think of yourself as some sort of an artist. Do those kinds of visualizations. Read about them. The literature is out there for people to learn how to visualize, how to meditate. There is so much information out there. In fact, I was on a plane recently and I was amazed when I plugged in those little earphones, right before you take off, that there was a kind of meditation tape going on. A woman was saying, "Take five deep breaths - take a deep breath. Hold it five seconds. Exhale. Now imagine that your shoulders are getting calm, that your arms are getting calm, that you're now going to be able to relax in your seat." This kind of thing is now almost mainstream. I would encourage anyone to try and find those resources.

I think that there's a tremendous link between what goes on emotionally and what happens to your body, in terms of cancer. I would so strongly suggest that anyone who is diagnosed with breast cancer understand that it's a little bump in the road. It's a bump. It's unpleasant. It's there. You deal with it. But you understand that this is a way to discover what's been going on that might have added to this. Find that out and make sure that you take care, that you don't allow that to happen again. Everybody has loss in their life. Everyone has grief. But it does not mean that you lose hope, that you lose the reason for living, that you despair.

It's a perfectly delightful thing to be a survivor. Survivors have wonderful personalities, they really do, I mean, they know the price of things. People have said to me, "Why do you call your book <u>The Immune Spirit</u>?" I said, it's really because your spirit has to be immune to these things that can come along and clobber you. That is the most important immunity you have to have, that of your spirit.

Dr. O. Carl Simonton

Oncologist

The father of modern medicine, William Osler, had two famous sayings: "Don't tell me what kind of disease the patient has. Tell me what kind of patient has the disease." A number of his quotes are quite famous. But another one of my favorites of his is, speaking of pulmonary tuberculosis, he said: "Care of the person with tuberculosis depends more on what they have in their head than what they have in their chest."

Our mind is central in our health. It's central. It's probably the most important single factor. And that is so far away from the current medical thought - which is that the mind and the emotions have no significant impact on physical health. Which is such a stupid concept. How we could maintain such ignorance over the years, and maintain it - in spite of the huge amount of evidence that's coming out day after day. To me, the only thing that reasonably explains it is our attachment to our way of thinking. We don't want to embrace ideas that uproot old ideas.

I started this because it was clear to me that a central problem in the patients I was addressing had to do with the mind and emotions. Now, I didn't understand that that had such a profound impact on the disease itself. But, I could see how it impacted the quality of treatment and what was going on. So, I began to investigate that - the role of hopelessness and how you address emotional issues in patients. Once I started into that area - wow, it was mind-boggling. And then I started to read. I found there had been a huge amount of work done in this area, and the more I read - it was while I was in Germany that my German director came across this quote from Hippocrates.

The quote was about the "brain" and was this: "From it comes all of our joy, happiness and all of our pain and suffering, as well as our other emotions, come from the brain." The way that statement tends to be made from Buddhist thought, which has studied consciousness for the past 2,500 years - they say from the mind, not from the brain. But, in Hippocrates' day they didn't use the concept of the mind, but he said "from the brain."

I started to address the mind, emotions, and issues of the human spirit, as part of my practice of medicine. It was Prendergast, who was the past President of the American Cancer Society, who in the 1950s said, "Who of us, in treating cancer, have not seen a person who was treated for breast cancer who was free of disease for twenty years? Then, with the death of a son in the war or infidelity of a daughter-in-law, or a financial downturn, then caused a flare up of their disease." This says that we cannot, as thinking individuals, we cannot ignore the relationship between these traumas and the flare up of disease in people who have been free of disease for a long period of time. And, he made the request that we widen our research to look at the role of the mind in the development and course of disease. This was in his presidential address to the American Cancer Society in the 1950s. I think 1956, and it's quoted in my book Getting Well Again.

The work of people like Kloeffer: Kloeffer was a Professor of Psychiatry at UCLA, and his work was around the placebo effect. He has a tremendous understanding of the role of belief in the placebo effect, and so he was involved in this clinical trial again in the 50s. Where this person was close to death, he received Probiocin, which was considered a worthless treatment. But, they were doing a clinical trial to prove it, and the guy went from near death to return to work. Dramatic recovery, lung metastasis, extensive disease, and then he got worse. Kloeffer said it's not the Probiocin that is related to his recovery, but his belief in the Probiocin, and we have an opportunity to prove it. So they structured a lie, telling him there had been an error and it had now been corrected. They were getting the new double-strength Probiocin being air freighted in. Kept him in the state of anticipation. He was equally close to death again, requiring oxygen at rest, having extensive pulmonary metastasis with fluid in his lungs, as well as large visible masses. They gave him, with much fanfare, the "new" Probiocin that had finally arrived. With much fanfare, they gave him injections of sterile water. The cancer went away faster with the sterile water than it had with the Probiocin. He went back to work and was doing well until a few months later. There was an article that came out stating that "Probiocin has now been proven to be of no value in the treatment of cancer," to which he responded by re-entering comatose - going to the emergency room and dying without regaining consciousness.

It is my deep belief that the rise of cancer is because we're experiencing more stress - and the primary stress we're experiencing is emotional distress - without good methods of relieving the distress. It's been shown over and over again that this drives our bodies' healing systems in the direction of illness and premature death. It's not even being looked at - not seriously being looked at anywhere in the world. It's clear that this is a huge factor, and I think it's the largest single factor in illness.

It isn't being looked at because we see what we believe; we don't believe what we see. Number one is we tend to be attached to our old way of thinking and this is a hugely different way of thinking. That goes on everywhere in the culture. If you have a paradigm shift, such as this, the result would be you would have a huge shift of power. Currently, physicians are not knowledgeable about the mind - not knowledgeable about consciousness. So the people that are knowledgeable and are able to address such issues, would have more power and the current physicians would have less. It's a huge power shift and with that comes a huge financial shift. So, you have these three areas. Number one, our attachment to our way of thinking that is culture-wide, that's everywhere. Then, we have protection of power. And then protection of income, which is from the medical profession. Also, from the pharmaceutical industry, because if we begin to acknowledge the tremendous self-healing power that we all possess, then we aren't going to need an eight feet high, twelve feet long, cold remedy section in our supermarkets.

Lewis Thomas, the renowned oncologist who was the head of Sloane Kettering, said one of the biggest tragedies that has happened in America is lack of respect for self-healing powers - for the powers of the body to heal itself. And we see this exemplified by the enlarging sections in our supermarkets devoted to cold remedies. We don't respect that our bodies can make a huge difference as far as developing an illness or not.

Counseling the person with a serious illness, we need to

focus on what's right with them, not what's wrong with them. So, the way we do that is to begin by having them focus on the many things that bring them a sense of joy and deep fulfillment. We have them list at least five, and begin to engage more in those activities that bring them joy. Then we address the things that interfere with that, and when they interfere. So that's the basic way that we approach the work.

Look at the things that bring you joy, and do more of those things. Then, we will begin to talk about other things, such as; we're healthy by nature. We're healthy by nature and what you're wanting your body to do is to get back to doing what it has done so well, for so many years - and that is to recognize, identify, transform and eliminate cancer cells.

And why did you get sick in the first place? What was the message, what was the meaning of illness and for this? The first place - this is clearly pointed out is in the Vedic teachings out of India from about seven thousand years ago where they said that illness is a signal, a signal that something is out of balance, something is out of whack. As we pay attention to that and adjust those issues, then number one, our lives will become richer and our health improves. So that illness, as Elida Evans wrote in her wonderful book that published in the 1920s, she said that cancer is a signpost in the road of life, calling out for change. But it's not punishment; it's a signal that something that we are doing is bad for us. And the message is to pay attention to that and begin to adjust that - to know that as we adjust that appropriately, our lives will become richer.

In 1972, I'd just been doing this work for about a year, and I had this young man in the military, who was, I think, eighteen or nineteen. He told me, "When I got my diagnosis (he had a non-Hodgkin's lymphoma) I felt euphoric, I felt elated, happy. Of course." he said, "I didn't tell anyone, because they would think I was crazy." So, I began to speak to him about why, because clearly, I now understand that our emotions are always appropriate to our beliefs. See, we have fear of cancer because of what we believe that means - both what the diagnosis means, what treatment we'll need to have and what that means - so obviously this young man had a very different framework for seeing this. Because this is the basis of cognitive therapies. We're not upset by things, but by the view we take of them. So, my job then was to determine what his view was. And it turns out that he had joined the Air Force when I was in charge of cancer treatment for western United States for the Air Force. He said, "I joined the Air Force to get back at my parents because they were always telling me what to do. I always had to come home at a certain time, so I thought to myself, 'I'll show them, I'll join the military.'" So he joined the military and instead of having parents and a few other people telling him what to do, he now had virtually everyone telling him what to do. And he said, "I couldn't even cry myself to sleep at night," because he was in barracks with a lot of other guys - so he couldn't even cry, couldn't even grieve what was going on.

And so when he got his diagnosis, he thought, aha, I'll get out, so he felt excited and elated. What he didn't understand is that in the military, when this situation arises, we have what's called TDRL – Temporary Duty Retirement List. And so you're taken from active duty and put on TDRL, which means now you have to be evaluated every three months or every so often. If you get well enough to return to active duty, you're back in active duty. And in order to stay on TDRL you have to stay sick, so I mean he was caught. But again, he had no idea of that. He thought, "I have cancer, I'll get out," so again, it depends again on our beliefs about the disease.

Since then, I've experienced a lot of different experiences around the diagnosis, so certainly the most common is fear - because those are the beliefs that most commonly were produced, and fear is what most people have. However, the emotional response is always appropriate to the beliefs about the event, not to the event - but to the beliefs about the event. And there can be a huge variation, as I stated in this case.

It's important that we develop strength in our beliefs in our body's ability to heal itself. So we need to imagine it working in a very competent way, that's number one. Number two; we need to develop effective ways in thinking about all the treatments that we're taking. So, whatever we're taking - the emotional work we're doing, the dietary changes that we're making, the traditional treatments that we're taking - it's important that anything we're doing, we need to see it as a friend and an ally. And then create healthier beliefs about cancer as a disease.

Again, most people don't realize that cancer is a weak disease, composed of weak, confused, deformed cells. When I tell most people that a cancer cell has never been demonstrated to attack a normal cell, they find that hard to believe. But I came from studying cell biology, so this is part of why things didn't make sense to me - because that information seemed to be ignored. So, if we're dealing with a disease composed of weak, confused, deformed cells that are killing us, why is that happening? And most of the early work showed that we get an increased outpouring of stress hormones - because we're staying in a distressed state that interferes with our body's healing mechanisms and increases the carcinogens. So, we get more cancer cells produced in response to the same cancer-causing agents.

The answer to that is a different state of mind. Then when we begin to bring in more calm, peacefulness, in the direction of joy and happiness, then you get an increase in our bodies' healing mechanisms - whether you're talking about the chemicals, or the neuroendocrine components or the immune components. All of them move in the direction of health when we engage in, or when we're focused primarily on, the emotions of peacefulness, joy and happiness.

So that's what we're going for; I develop healthier beliefs, since our emotions are always appropriate to our beliefs. As I develop healthier beliefs about my body's ability to heal itself, healthier beliefs about the treatments that I'm taking, everything that I'm doing to enhance my health, and healthier beliefs about cancer as a disease - then that's going to influence my overall emotional response every time I am reminded that I have cancer. So if I have unhealthy beliefs, then I'm going to experience emotional distress every time I'm reminded. If I have healthier beliefs I'm going to be more calm when I'm reminded. And then, it's important to pay attention to what the message is. What is the meaning? According to most of the literature, the message of illness is a compassionate message. The message is to do more of those things that bring you joy, more of those things that bring you joy and deep fulfillment, and do less of those things that cause you pain.

As an oncologist, I know how oncologists are trained. I

know how physicians are trained. We're not trained to understand consciousness. We're not trained to understand the role of the mind in health. So, if we're not trained to that, how are we going to help people do that? We're not trained to do it. This is not a new problem. This is a problem that's going on everywhere because Western medicine is the model for world medicine. It's a problem everywhere.

When I was in training, there was a huge difference in the incidents of cancer of the prostate in American men versus Japanese men. In American men, the statistics are: "Approximately fifty percent of men over fifty have cancer of the prostate. And nearly sixty percent of the men over sixty, seventy percent over seventy, so it's easy to remember". Japan, much less. So it was always argued back and forth: Is it the fish they eat? Or, it's the…and, I said when I got into this work, "If we knew the sexual habits of the Japanese man. Therein lies the answer to this issue." I had no way of understanding the sexual habits of Japanese men or no access to this information. Well, as I started working in Japan, my translator gave me two books to read. One of them was called <u>The Chrysanthemum And The Sword</u>, and it's considered the best description from a Westerner of Japanese life. It says that the sexual habits of the Japanese male pre-World War II and post-World War II are the differences between night and day. The difference between Japanese sexual habits and Western sexual habits are as different as night and day. They went into specifics about what the differences were. But this was the first time I was reading exactly what I had hypothesized thirty years ago.

This is very gratifying to see how this plays out. Because

there was no real sexual frustration in the Japanese male. Now there is, and I would assume that the cancer of the prostate has come up significantly. Ours is still as high as it used to be.

Breast cancer is another disease I have looked at a lot. I think in young women, in women under, say fifty, the biggest underlying issue is role conflict. If you take cultures where there is virtually no role conflict - and I had an opportunity to do this with the Native American Indian population. With the Native American Indian population and prior to say 1950, it was very common for Native American women to stay on the reservation. When they stayed on the reservation, their role was homemaker, period. As they started to move and the incidents of breast cancer rose - breast cancer before 1950 was virtually unheard of in Native American Indians - as they began to become more Westernized and work off the reservation and were conflicted about role conflict, the incidents of breast cancer began to rise. So that's one place that I saw this. In older women, I'm not sure. But in younger women, it's role conflict and sexual identity issues. You listen to American women, and they're conflicted about working outside the home and caring for the children. There's huge conflict around that.

Resolving their internal conflict over their appropriate roles, you can see what a huge issue this is, this issue of role conflict. It's easy to discover for ourselves if we're interested, because all I need to do is pay attention to my own emotional guidance system. When I'm feeling neutral, that's good for my health. Joy, happiness all those things are good. When I am in distress, regardless of the form of distress, that's bad for my health and the longer I stay there, the more frequently I go there. As I do this, the more I'm secreting these unhealthy compounds driving my healing system in the direction of illness and death. That's one of the principle ways we're taught to deal with ourselves. According to most authorities in this area, in the mind body area, emotional distress always precedes physical illness.

We want to become more aware of our emotional distress, but we need - as we become more aware of our emotional distress - to know what to do about it. Because to simply be more aware of it would decrease our quality of life. It's not a blessing if I'm more aware of my distress, but I don't know what to do about it.

The solutions are so simple. According to one of the most simple processes for dealing with distress when it comes up is - most people want to go from distress to joy - is realizing going from distress to joy doesn't work effectively. The thing that we can do is to incrementally move up the scale. And the way that we're taught to do that is to think about one of those things that bring us joy and deep fulfillment. Hold that thought for only thirty seconds, a short amount of time, then think about a second such thought, and hold that for thirty seconds, then think about a third. Now in a minute and a half, they say in general, you at least will have moved up very significantly where you can tell the difference. And so you gain competency in using this very simple process.

It's a lot like this: we have it all round us, count your blessings, pay attention to the things that you appreciate and love. And one of my favorite things to think about is that little dog that was running around here, because she's - I mean if she were allowed - she'd be either under the coffee table or at my feet right now. Because when I'm home, she's always around because she knows that I love her and it's such a nourishing, nurturing relationship. Pets are excellent at helping people focus on the things that bring them joy.

http://www.simontoncenter.com/

Thomas Lodi, M.D.

Founder
Oasis for Healing

I dropped out of school at nineteen. I was at UCLA and I dropped out and moved to India. I came back to the U.S. and pursued psychology and got a graduate degree in psychology, as a clinical psychologist. I worked for a couple years and then found that I just didn't know enough. There were too many areas of physiology and pathology that I didn't understand. I didn't understand the effect certain medications had on people. So I wound up going to medical school. My journey was a spirit/mind/body journey into all this.

I did my training, my internship and residency, in Internal Medicine at Columbia University in New York. I wound up practicing for about ten years as an internist in ICUs and CCUs and internal medicine, urgent cares. I saw that it doesn't work. It's real good as a band-aid, but it just doesn't work. So, I wound up at that point going around the world to different countries and learning a little bit of what I could from Japan, around the U.S., Mexico, different practitioners.

Then I went and started practicing in New York, using all that I had learned. It finally happened that I began to narrow the focus onto oncology, what I've come to call integrative oncology. I use a little bit of conventional medicine, though modified. I use botanical medicine. I use oxidative medicine. I do all those sorts of things. But the foundation of what I do is teaching people how to change their lives.

We don't catch health and neither do we catch disease. We earn either. It's what we earn. The old saying that we dig our graves with our teeth is true, with every bite we take. Just as we have new skin every six weeks, we have new rods and cones in our eyes every forty eight hours, we have new lining in our colon every three days, new livers every four to six months, and we have a new body every ten to twelve months. So, if we have a condition a year ago and we have it today, it's because we're continuing to produce it. We need to understand that. It's very important to understand that we are dynamic processes of becoming.

So you can stop at any moment, what you're doing, and change what you're feeding this machine - and this machine will do what it wants to do, what it needs to do, what it is designed to do. That is to heal and grow. That's what it was designed to do.

Vaccination is actually the inoculation of disease. We're putting in viral protocols. We're putting in live viruses. It's an insane concept to believe it could be of any benefit. We get immunization by being exposed to real life. We get the measles. You only get them once. Chicken pox, you only get them once. The main thing to do is, for healthcare, is to preserve your immune system, preserve your vitality and get exposed. Why do we use colostrum from cows? Because down in the dirt, they're dirty. They have feces in their mouths. Their immune system is constantly being challenged so it's very powerful. So we use their immunity. Eight hundred animals drink out of the same watering hole in the jungle and they don't get sick. The point is to get that exposure. You don't need the inoculation of diseases.

Our immunity is failing. Our colons are full of feces. We

have five feet of colon. We don't empty that once a day like we should. Five feet of it. If you don't, you're going to continue to absorb those toxins. Those toxins are absorbed straight up to the liver.

Because there's no nutrition in the food, or very little, there's always a hunger, this hidden hunger. They just finished two pizzas and they're still hungry. They're at the buffet and they're on their eighth plate and they're still not satisfied. The reason why we're not satisfied is because there're no nutrients there. Eating is designed to nourish the organism. What we're doing is we're using it to masturbate our tongues. That's what we're doing. That's our reward. Our reward is obesity coupled with malnutrition. Then if you consider the fact that we're breathing in toxins and we're also exposed to electromagnetic things, there's no way on earth that we could possibly not get cancer. I'm surprised we make it to the age of thirty.

The immune system is the department of defense and the department of maintenance. When it's overwhelmed with maintenance requirements, basically our defense goes on hold. So a full colon, continually eating bad foods…..our immune system, sixty to seventy percent of our immune system is in our gastrointestinal tract. So it's continually working and working, and it gets exhausted. It gets overwhelmed. Now you get exposed to something that requires an immune response and you just don't have it. You're just not capable of it. When you get a number of those assaults, which we have through the vaccinations and all that… it's amazing that we make it as far as we do. It's kind of like George Burns smoking cigars made it to a hundred. In spite of that he made it to a hundred. That's how incredible a system we have. But look at him, when he grew up there was only organic food. There was fresh air.

Diseases are the shadows of health. They're ephemeral. Shadows aren't real. They kind of move here and there, depending on what's blocking them. But the blockage is to health. Health is the light and darkness is disease. If you look at that, the only place you're going to have darkness is where there's a shadow, which is an obstruction. So the absence of light is darkness. The absence of health is disease. It's not the other way around.

Our bodies, as does all of nature, are designed to regenerate, rejuvenate and procreate. That's it. That's the imperative of nature. You pick a plant; you pick a few leaves and then there are ten more leaves. You pick an apple; there are eight more apples. That's the way it is. You cut your arm; it heals. Nature is in the state of becoming and growing and procreating. That's what nature does, just as water rolls downhill. It's as natural as that.

The only way that stops is if you put impediments. That's what we do. We continually put impediments to that. It works around it. Just like water will go around the one boulder. But if you get enough boulders and all that, you eventually block it. That's what happens.

It's very simple. We have to undo, stop doing, stop eating. Fasting, cleanse, allow the body…because you're not healing when you're eating and digesting. You can't heal. You only heal when you're not eating. So you heal, in like, the last couple hours of sleep because you've finally emptied your GI tract. So going to bed full is a real terrible thing because you're not going to get much healing done.

Healing is what will happen if you stop and start fasting and then cleanse. That has a lot to do with healing. You've got to eat proper foods. You've got to eat human food. Human food is plants.

Healing comes from the same place disease comes from - it's part of nature. All we can do is make sure that your body is getting what it needs and it will heal. It's not me. It's God. It's the Universe. It's the way it is. It's the nature of nature to heal. I'm going to help you remove your impediments. Once you remove your impediments, healing will happen. It's not something I do. You can't purchase a cure, but you can earn your health. You can't purchase a cure, but you can earn your health. It's a very important concept.

I had a stage four lung cancer man that was told he had three weeks to live. In five weeks, he was dancing outside at the clinic. He had a clean CAT scan. Another woman who had breast cancer that had metastasized to most of her lungs, she couldn't breathe without the help of oxygen. She couldn't bathe herself or take care of herself, couldn't go to the toilet - and within eight weeks, she was jogging to our clinic and her husband was driving the car behind her. Those are just two stories; they keep happening.

It's a comprehensive approach. Stop making cancer, target and eliminate the cancer without harming the person, and stimulate and enhance the immune system. If you do all three of those things at once....

You want to eat right, live right. Make your body alkaline.

It's just plant material. Raw, unprocessed plant material. It doesn't mean you just sit around chewing on alfalfa leaves. But you can make wonderful dishes. You can use dehydrators. Make sure that the food is alive. If you're going to eat an animal, eat that animal alive. That's how carnivores do it. Carnivores don't eat dead animals. So if you want to eat an animal, eat it alive, or freshly dead. I just say that because I know you're not going to do it. What I'm really saying is we're not designed to eat animals. We're designed to eat plants. We are vegetarians. That's what our makeup is. If you look at our saliva to our jaws to everything, that's the way we are.

So when you eat the plants, when they're alive, they still have that bioelectric charge, which is vitality. We need that. We need that bioelectric charge because that's what is - from the sun to the plants to the animals to us. If you get an animal, you're getting it secondhand. So, we really need to get it firsthand from the plants. So you get that energy, you get that electricity, you get that life. That's what life is. Mary Shelley, when she wrote Frankenstein, knew that you need electricity. She was trying to get electricity into him. If you're flat-lined in the ER, we give you electricity. That bioelectric charge, which is the carrier of chi, the carrier of qi, the prana, that's the vitality that enlivens the flesh. You've got to get that from a live plant. If you cook the plant, it's dead. The thing is, we're not necrophages. We shouldn't eat dead material. We need to eat live material.

All plants, nuts, seeds, roots are our food. And fruit, of course. Lots of fruit is our natural diet. When we eat that way we come alive, diseases don't happen.

The first step is to go out and purchase a lot of organic green vegetables. Make sure you have like kale, dandelion, spinach, broccoli, cucumber, celery, maybe a lemon to take away the bitterness and then a few green apples. You don't want to make it too sweet. You put that all together. You juice it. Just do that for twenty-one days. Get your colon clean. Do an enema. Do whatever you can to clean your colon, or colonics. And just drink four, five, six quarts a day. Just flood your body. What'll happen is you don't have to worry about not being nourished, because in one jar of juice you're getting this many vegetables, just the fiber is removed. So you're getting actually more nourishment in one jar than the average American gets in a year, two years. So you're getting well nourished, and you're flooding your body with chlorophyll, which has got magnesium, which is alkalinizing. You will just come alive. Your brain will clear up. Your energy will clear up. Everything improves, from your ability to focus to your libido.

http://www.anoasisofhealing.com/

Anna Wiedeler

Inspirationalist

I was diagnosed with breast cancer in 1997 or '98 - one of those. And in 2001, I was diagnosed with metastasis breast cancer. I remember getting the phone call from the surgeon at ten o'clock at night. I was alone at home and she called me to say, "I have bad news for you. The pathology came back and you have cancer." I received it in a very calm way, as if time stood still. And what was interesting as I sat there quite numb in my chair - and one of the first things that came clearly to me - was literally a voice inside my head. Not that I heard it, but a knowing that said, "Your love of self and life and not fighting breast cancer will heal you." And, I knew kind of theoretically what that meant, because I really knew my patterns of self-destructive things and self-rejection and so forth. But what it meant really to put that into practice, I had trouble with.

Then of course, after I got the news - the barrage of the medical system, the urgency to rush you into immediate action - that this is life threatening and so forth, I totally got swept up in that field of energy, literally! Because medicine comes from the understanding that it's this formidable, deadly opponent you have and you better go and kill it. And from my background, I'm a holistic practitioner; I was really in conflict with that.

So I tried to get my bearings, but I really was swept up right away. I received a lumpectomy within a week and unfortunately in that time, they still did radical lymph node removal and so forth. So, I went through that. However, I was glad I recovered quite fast from the surgery. Then, I was urged tremendously to undergo chemotherapy and radiation, which I refused. I just couldn't get myself to - it was against all my belief system, against all my belief system. What I did then, I researched a lot of alternative things and ended up for about a year self-injecting myself with a substance called 714X, which is an immune system and lymph booster. However, in my fear, there was a real fear in me that I had ducked something. Like I had evaded something. I always had that little fear in the background - it will come back, it will come back, it will come back. And not because I didn't think what I was doing wasn't working, but I had chickened out of facing the real therapy, which was chemotherapy.

It took about two or three years, or I think four, until the recurrence happened. And at the time, what preceded it was we renovated the house and my anger - my resentment with the drama that went on with the process - I think really was what brought on the discord in me again. Because, of course, I also started looking at what is it in my life that I have to change. Nothing is as good as a teacher, as you know, as a possibly terminal disease - so you clean up your act quickly.

I found some more lumps again. And I ended up actually then having to look at chemotherapy because now it was systemic. It was not a local event anymore. I also had forgotten that right after my lumpectomy, within six months, I had learned that at the lumpectomy my margins weren't clear. But, I still didn't want to get any further things done; however, within six months I had more lumps in my breast. I opted for a radical mastectomy and reconstruction. All through that time I also looked at my tremendous fears and issues I have with the medical field. Because somehow I polarized myself to believe that the ones in the white coats were the bad guys and we are the alternative part - we're the good guys. And here I was now, in my camp, and the things didn't work. So when I was diagnosed, then with metastasis breast cancer, I really knew I might have to do something a bit more drastic. And, I also knew it was time. And by that time, four years later, I was ready to say, "Okay, I can do chemo."

And I started doing chemo. It was actually, by far, less brutal then I had anticipated it. I lost all my hair, which was a big issue; however, I refused to wear a wig. So I went bald for quite a while. And through it all, though, I never really felt bad. I think my own self-care, my nutritional things, my activity, my physical exercise always gave me enough energy to keep plowing on, so even when I was on chemo, I would rollerblade. I would go running. It was amazing how much energy I had.

I would have acupuncture treatments, I would exchange with my colleagues, I'd practice holistic bodywork, zero balancing. I would receive sessions like that. I would really look at my nutrition - I would reduce sugar, eat wholesome foods, drop alcohol and those kinds of things. I really started - and I always had in the back of my mind "your love of self and your love of life" - trying to find a better balance in my life. This was in terms of what would be the self-loving thing to do now, to have a glass of wine, or to not have one. So I didn't make rules. I basically said, when I wanted a glass of wine, "Is this to reduce my stress, or is this to enjoy myself even more?" So I know the difference - when I do something to avoid something, or when I do something to enhance something. And so, I think over these eight or nine years, it sounds now so level-headed. It now sounds that I always knew what I wanted.

This experience was literally purgatory. It was difficult. It was wrenching. What I put myself through, and people through, was arduous.

So, some of the things that I learned through my treatment were - I read it in a manual-book, where the author said, "Cancer is fear, and unless you deal with fear, you're missing the point so to speak." And once I started looking at fear being the opposite of love, I started looking at where are my fears? I started looking at what are my fears of? Really the medical system, of the doctors - I realized, really my fear of authority. Speaking against what they wanted me to do, denying what they want me to pursue, and in that process of selecting what doctor works for me, I really learned to speak up and speak my mind. And a lot of it went with a lot of tears and a lot of drama. But, I have to say by now I am really well with physicians, and I've found a wonderful oncologist who literally supports me through everything I go through. He doesn't cajole, he doesn't push, he offers. He says, "Anna, I'm an oncologist, this is what I do, this is what I have to offer, here is what my opinion is…and then he leaves it, and he always says, "Whatever you want to do, look at yourself."

He said, "You're doing well. How can I not support you in what you're doing because you're doing well?" So, I now am under the care of a good oncologist who really is part of my team and is not the leader. I am the team leader. That is very clear, and he has enough self-esteem to not need to tell me who the boss is. And that is wonderful; Peter is a wonderful, wonderful partner in my healing journey. And I'm also under the care of a classical homeopath, where I'm being treated constitutionally, literally for those qualities of my personality that are fearful. You know, the perfectionist, critic that is coming always from fear, saying that it's not good enough - I'm not good enough, and so forth.

So when I look back, yes, I've been diagnosed nine years ago with cancer; I think I had cancerous behavior since I was a child. When I look at....from where we learn our beliefs? How do we take life, how do we understand ourselves? That foundation is learned in childhood, how we take life and life's stresses, interpret it and see ourselves. And I think I made, very early on, the decision that I'm all by myself and I'm all alone - coming from an alcoholic family, you figure it out for yourself. My father was a loving, wonderful man, but he was an alcoholic. And trusting - keeping his word was not one of his strengths when he was on booze. So, there were some real trust issues and faith issues with him. And being brought up Catholic where God the Father is the one you need to surrender to - or you need to trust or you believe in. I think in a young mind, parents are God, and I also never trusted some higher power - because, you know you have to do it in the end by yourself. And I think that, in itself, is a stressful way to live, because you run into your own limits quite a lot.

So for me, recovering from cancer or healing from cancer really has been more or less a spiritual journey - seeing what does surrender mean? What is my role of actively taking responsibility? What defines my role of letting go? And that is really where I am today. What do I need to do? Yes, if medicine has come up with the best medicine has to offer, why put that down? So, I have basically come full circle. I now would never turn away something because it comes from the traditional field. Because I've seen that with one's belief, and also seeing that the physicians have good intent, physicians also lose family members to cancer. So it's like - I had this really strange idea of physicians somehow. So I see that also they want the best for me and ultimately, yes, I'm the one who calls the shots. Over those nine years, I've become very self-reliant, trusting the decisions I make. I realize at some point I will not extend my life one second longer when my time is up.

So, if I do this therapy or that therapy, if I go on this road or that road, I don't think it will matter in the end. I really don't think so. I think for whom, what's the phrase, the bell tolls - it's time to go. And not to look then at whether I died from cancer or not - it is really irrelevant. What is important is what have I done with the time that I was alive? And I realize that cancer is not so much a particular set of symptoms that you have. It's a mental idea of terrific things, horrific things. And it literally is like a minefield that you get swept up in. It's terror that you get pulled into. All really what we have to do is get out of fear and we get out of what I call "cancering."

Now does that mean that a fearless person does not, will not ever get cancer? I don't dare to make those kinds of statements, but I do know that we now know that every thought immediately is translated into physiology and physiological reaction. So I do know when loving thoughts are thought, the body is thriving. When fearful thoughts are engaged, the body suffers.

So my intention really is to be as relaxed, as hopeful, as loving as possible - to see the good. Is that easy all the time? No, but without lying, I can really say today that cancer was certainly not the best thing that happened to me. That would be an outright lie. However, I would not want to be the person I was before I got diagnosed. That is a huge difference, and I like who I have become. I like my life. Saying yes to myself has made it much more sweet, much more peaceful. So that has been the biggest change - the opportunity - that cancer can give oneself. It's an opportunity.

The redeeming value of looking at it as an opportunity… See, I don't dare to say I know how to cure cancer, but I do know how to deal with my fears. That is something I know I can face. So what it does do? It empowers me to be active in my life, in my healing, because I do know that letting go of fear is healing. When we look at the word health, healing, it comes from the Anglo-Saxon word "hal," which means to make whole. To become whole - and so healing is to make whole, to become whole - which I equate with letting go of fear and recognizing who we are - body, mind and spirit. We are divine. We are made in the likeness and image of the Divine. And fear is a denial of that. And so if I claim and connect with that knowing of who I am, that certainly puts me into a totally different space than feeling like a little human worm that had the bad luck of being, you know, hit by an incurable disease and there's no way out. So I chose to look at it as my opportunity to become more than I ever thought I would.

There is a limited time in this body, in this space suit, and within that time I would like to fulfill the purpose for which I came, which is to become conscious of who I am. That, I think, really is the purpose of life. What does it mean to be human? Who we are is really the central question. And the central question in a disease is who am I?

A victim, or am I the creator of my life? So that for me has been tremendously empowering.

I really understand in that way, whether one gets a cold or high-blood pressure or cancer, the ideology is not different. I think why one develops cancer and another one gets this or that, I think there's also a lot of one's internal experience. After all, life is a mystery. One's soul journey is not to be fully understood because otherwise you would miss the lessons, right?

I think the reason for that is multi-faceted. One is always where do we direct our attention? I'm not of any particular religion, but I loved what Jesus said, resist no evil. Whatever we fight gets more. Look at the war on drugs – we have more junkies than ever before, and the war on drugs hasn't led to anything but more druggies and more crime around it. So the war on cancer will produce more cancer. Because whatever we focus on - for example, right after being diagnosed you become sensitized - you go to the post office, and you didn't think of your stuff, and there was this big sign "Stamp out breast cancer." So that was in my face again. Every woman's glossy you look through - how to do your breast exam, how to check, how to look for - and it may sound very radical, and I think it may produce medical rage when I say this, but I believe self exams cause more breast cancer than they prevent. The law: Seek and you shall find. Which woman will examine her breast lovingly and say, "Oh, do I find something new?" Isn't there an element of fear and anxiety, what she could detect? And when she detects something, she's going to go for the needle. And then, they'll do this and that - and the fear increases, and all that goes with that. Monthly now, I look for trouble in my body. I mean do you take a dental mirror every month and you look for trouble in your teeth? No, you don't. The next thing is now we are supposed to look every year for trouble in our intestines.

I really believe that as long as we see our body as a source of possible betrayal, and falling apart, we will create those. Because, after all, it is our beliefs in our minds that create our reality. And if I believe in a body that is susceptible to invaders, that is susceptible to diseases - where some enemy comes out of the woodwork to get me - that, I think, is terror. And that's the war on terror that I think is acting out also in the world. We need to face our fear, regardless of what fear that is. So that is one aspect, I think what we have done to the planet environmentally - what we drink, eat, breath - is where I think our politicians should be held accountable. And that in and of itself is also incomplete. We should be held accountable. Why don't we demand that? Clean air, clean water, clean whatever - is my right. Rather than having to go and buy bottled water. Next thing is, you buy bottled air. Though I have to say I have good hope that we are at a turning point, because I do see it everywhere and I look for that.

What I have seen is that when you go to any drug store, you get ready for the flu season. Nobody has had the flu, the flu hasn't arrived yet, but you get ready - and I think that in itself is mass hypnosis. When you go to classes... and teachers, you know when somebody says, "Don't hug me, or don't give me a hand because I've got a cold?" It is this belief that I could be susceptible to something. I truly have never gotten the flu from anybody because I don't take anybody else's germs. Even though they are with me, I don't have an issue with them. My body can handle them. I had this thing about being afraid of being around cancer, and that's of course, what I got. We get what we are afraid of and what we attract. Now many people may say, "Well when I was diagnosed, I certainly wasn't afraid of anything," and I would say, "Well, just look. You may not have been afraid of cancer, but you may have been afraid, or covering up or not dealing with some deeper issue, that you were afraid to bring up to the surface. Otherwise you wouldn't have cancer." It is that, so cancer, in and of itself, has that insidious onset. Nobody blares out and suddenly gets this huge tumor - that's very rare - but it comes over years, and it's just been sitting there. That's just what we do with our emotions and our unresolved business and resentments and grievances.

With the wisdom that I've gained now, what I would do differently is not let myself be rushed, bullied into doing anything. I would say, "You know what, if that's what I've got, this is not a matter of life and death. It isn't. Whether a lumpectomy is being done today or in a week, or in two weeks, doesn't make any difference." I would not let my lymph nodes be removed. But other than that, I could not change what I've done, because that all added up to who I have become. So even in that sense, the lumpectomy, the lymph nodes removal, the mastectomy, all those things, haven't been wrong because each one was part and parcel of my healing journey. So if I were to talk to anybody, I would always say, "What feels right to you? What gives you the greatest sense of optimism, hope and healing? That's what you need to follow." If you need to combine this with that, go for it. If you need to deny that, but only want that, go for it. If you want to go the alternative route, go for it. If you want to go and see the guru in Brazil, go for it. Whatever brings you to the next step of ease, because really healing is leaving dis-ease behind, and learning to go the path of ease. That really is my one and only message, and nobody knows it for you, but you. You know what's right for you.

Nobody knows somebody else's soul path. If there was something in their experience to be experienced - I liken it to this: Some people give up smoking and that's it. Other people try it fifteen times and have recurrences, so who am I to say what they need to do? We need to do what we need to do, and that's our own sacred journey. There is not one healing method for anything. There's only one's own self-sacred path of healing, and healing doesn't mean survival. Healing means how much closer to the recognition of who I am have I come? That is what healing is. So dying of cancer is not failure. I may die of cancer as a healed person and use cancer as my means to get out of this space suit. So, the other part of why so many people die of cancer, I think in this society, especially in the Western society, is that the taboo of dying is tremendous. So, you rarely meet a person who's heard that so and so died, who doesn't say, "Of what?" To leave this earth-suit behind just because you're done is not accepted. I mean death is the worst you can do to someone. I think there is no sacred way of leaving in this society. You need to have something to get out, to justify it, to say, "Well, it's better for him now." So I think that is one other reason why we choose, on an unconscious level, a way out. It's kind of blasphemy to say well, I was done! It's like walking out of a movie, and I think that's one of the reasons why we have these diseases. It's an acceptable way to say, "I'm done." It's certainly also a way to prepare people to say, "I'm leaving."

I meditate every day, and that has become my way of

living. I followed Stephen Levine's book <u>A Year to Live</u>, and I have cleaned up my act. There is not one person I don't talk to, or that I have grievances for; I am current with my unfinished business. There is no unfinished business. I do the best I can to live in the now and I have a file in my computer for when I die. I have arranged who gets what, where what goes, what I want to happen. I'm prepared. Even today, I'm current in my house; I don't have old stuff in there. I actually - when something new comes in, an old thing goes out - have that kind of revolving door. This whole hoarding or holding onto things, attachment to things, I live lightly. I try to do my best to live lightly and to also see the humor in it all. I've become - certainly in my looking at the fear that I had - like, gosh, the bottom line is always how do I look? Am I too fat? I mean, you know, if I look at some craziness in my treatment, one of the things I was delighted about going to chemo was I got thinner! You're talking about women's craziness about their slenderness. So it was a way to be thin.

So, to sum it up really I think, the ultimate message of cancer is to let go of the fear of death. If we haven't accepted our dying, we will always be afraid to live. So, I think as I confronted my own mortality and my dying and prepared for it, I got free to live - which is lighter than I've ever been. I can laugh about myself. There is nothing that I would hide from anybody else. I can tell you about my flaws, I know I'm a closet Martha Stewart, I know I have certain neurotics, but now I can laugh about them and I can say yes to them. I'm no longer ashamed of them, and I know I have the rest of my life you know, maybe, to improve on that, if necessary. Otherwise, people will have to live with me and Martha Stewart together!

Peter Heusser, M.D.

Anthroposophical Doctor
Switzerland

An anthroposophical clinic means it is actually a clinic working for integrative oncology or integrative medicine, specialized in the field of oncology. This means that we are all officially trained doctors here, but in addition - or in complementation of the conventional measures - we also use different therapies like herbs, minerals and music therapy, painting and movement therapy, called therapeutic eurhythmy. We also do counseling on spiritual and general life issues. What we actually try to do is to look at the patient in a holistic way, which means we include physical aspects, emotional aspects, cognitive aspects, spiritual aspects and social aspects. This is the whole thing and so we try to work on each level therapeutically, and that makes a kind of integrative, holistic, modern type of medicine, which of course includes conventional measures.

The human being is always a human being and not just a body, not just a physical bunch of materials. That's the reason why you always have to look at the whole issue. A tumor is not only caused by certain physical causes. It can also have other reasons. For example, your life-forces - which are expressed by your immune system - might be weak for certain reasons, for many reasons. Or, emotional issues might have bothered you for a long time, so this also has an influence on your biological situation, spiritual aspects, etc.

In the genesis of the tumor or of any illness, there are

many different possibilities. It's very well known that the tumor is not only caused by one singular agent on the physical level, but in addition to that, you can also say it's also caused by emotional, spiritual, and other aspects. Therefore, also in therapy, it's important to use a broader range of measures in order to treat the whole person - so that all these influences together can help to improve the outcome of the disease.

We have to learn to look at the human organism much more as being a totality, a whole thing, and to understand the functioning of the whole - instead of just looking at the parts as we're used to doing in the last two hundred years. And, I think this is a line of thinking that has to come about in the next decades.

Patients who are affected by tumors should not only go to the doctor and look at the tumor passively and say, "Hey doctor, fix me, take out this tumor." Yes, this should be done. But also, the human being, even much more so than the animals or plants, should focus on self-activity. This is on the mental level, spiritual level, emotional level and on also the level of life, biology. Therefore it is very important that the patients themselves try to contribute to healing in such a way that they, themselves, activate those means which fight against the tumor - in their organism, in their soul, in their spirit.

That's also one of the reasons why we address such questions with patients like lifestyle, nutrition, movement, emotional balance, spiritual aspects, the question of meaning and destiny. And, it's very important that the patient does not only look at the tumor alone, but this person also has a broad perspective, looking at himself or herself as a whole being. And in fact, I think that many,

many problems where patients have spiritual distress, for example, come from the fact that they are not used to living a spiritual life. Or, they're not used to having enough activity in their life. So, if they are confronted with such a thing as a tumor, they do not really know how to deal with that. And that's the reason why the help for the patient - to improve his coping with the disease - is so important. And, there are enough studies that show that the improvement of active coping also leads to a better outcome.

My personal impression is that through these two hundred years of reductionist science, this has led to a certain passivity - because a machine never has self-activity, not really, not like a plant that can reproduce itself, etc. I think to look at the human being differently - to look at what is really responsible for that inner self-activity - on the level of life, the level of soul, the level of spirit. That is one of the very important assignments for modern medicine in order to understand the whole human being better. I think if that changes - if the scientists themselves not only look at the human being as a machine, but as a living being, a soul being, a spiritual being - then I think the public also will more and more address these questions. If the doctors themselves only have the mechanistic approach to the human being, how should the broad public - which in a way looks up to the scientists - have another opinion? Therefore, I think that the striving of doctors to really understand what a human being is defines one of the most essential questions of today. You can feel that the public really wants to go in that direction.

People are very individual. Some people have many difficulties in looking at disease as a chance for something new, as a turning point. Those who manage that, something you hear very often is, "Since I have that disease, I realize how precious every moment of my life is, and I have learned much to distinguish between the essential and the non-essential. I have learned to take more earnestly my inner longings - and not only the demands from the outside or from career. I have learned to see that my essential, deeper questions are much more important for me than all these career questions, for example."

This is also something I can sometimes tell my patients to console them, to give them certain help emotionally. If they realize, for example, that if you have a heart attack and you die right away, you had no preparation at all. How much different it is to have had breast cancer, to have it removed, to be afraid maybe that it might come again - but to see that statistically you have years to come. Even if you would die, you have years to come. So you can prepare yourself.

Then you have a phase, maybe of years, of a much, much deeper and richer inner life than you would have had without the disease. So I do have some patients, especially women, who are more sensitive on this point - who tell me that thanks to their disease, they are actually living a more meaningful life. Taken from this perspective, diseases - in humanity disease will never cease to exist - illnesses do have a positive side, and they can contribute to the overall development in the human life. It's actually a process of becoming more mature, in the human sense. So Novalis, who was a famous German author, once said, "Human disease actually contributes to the overall human aim of human beings."

If doctors are really honest, they know that they can't make statements offering statistics, because what does three months mean? Three months means that maybe on the statistical average, people might have three months. But, you never know where in the statistic or in the variation your patients are. You might have a patient in front of you who will be freed from the disease and another one who will die in two weeks. How do you know? You never know. There are studies that show that doctors usually make a wrong judgment on that. They can't really predict that. Fortunately, they can't, because it's not their business to decide how long a patient has to live. They should do what they can. But a human being, of course, is not only physically determined, but may also be healing on other levels - including the spiritual one. The outcome is completely open, even if in a very dangerous situation. That's why I personally never tell the patients how many months I expect them to live.

I tell them, for example, "Listen, this is a very dangerous disease that you have, but it's very possible that you have a very good chance. We don't know. You should do everything that makes that possible." Then I think I'm really honest, too. I don't lie to the people, and I never make any promises. But I also tell them how open the situation really is - from a scientific side, even.

Every human being has his or her individual disease, even if it's the same type of cancer as someone else's. It's an individual type of cancer, and you always live in individual situations. You have your individual, very personal, destiny or karma, etc. So, you should always think that this might be like a message telling you that in some way you should maybe look at your life in a deeper sense. And then, as I said before, take all the measures you can, but deal also with other things. Have a spiritual trust, and then I think that's what you can do.

I sometimes compare that with a hike in the mountains. It has its ups and downs, and then all of a sudden it becomes steep when you do not expect it. But when you think, "Well now, I can't go on any longer," all of a sudden you have a beautiful panorama and there is a bench there where you can sit down. So, if you look at your life like a mountain hike to the top, and you take your step as you can in the moment, this is a good picture you can take with you. And, then you can also deal with your individual situation even better.

http://www.lukasklinik.ch/start/

Dr. Muralidhar

Ayurvedic Physician
India

If you look at the system of Ayurveda thousands of years ago, there were treatises written by great luminaries in Ayurveda. And if you look at those texts, they mention cancer and they have used the term abooda, which can be correlated to today's cancer. You will be surprised to see that this abooda has been categorized as an easily curable disease, in those times, an easily curable disease. But today the world, the entire medical profession, is struggling and doing more and more research in this field. Even though there is considerable progress, the results, the prognosis of the disease, is still limited. It has not achieved a safe area, as of today.

Ayurveda can help in treating cancer in two ways. One is to check the growth of cancer cells. And another line of treatment would be rejuvenation to cancer patients who have already undergone the trauma of chemotherapy or radiation therapy. So their tissues, their body tissues, and their minds, which are under quite a lot of stress and strain, can be rejuvenated to a certain extent.

Wherever it may be, the world has human beings of the same build. The main reason of the increase in cancer in the world today, we may put forth some important factors which are something considered like carcinogens, or cancer producing factors. One of them may be irregular or faulty food habits, and stress, and strain, and body and mind abuse. All these are already mentioned in the Ayurvedic texts - that some of these, when they are going to an unlimited state, they cause the growth of new or irregular shaped cells or infliction of cancer cells.

Even though toxins are getting inside the systems to all human beings in different degrees, only some people get inflicted by cancer. The reason could be that the immunity power or the difference mechanism in certain persons is very low. Once they start abusing the physical and mental suggestions of the body, they may get succumbed to this disease easier.

No medical system can give you a hundred percent cure prognosis treatment for cancer. It's always a risk. So, even though chemotherapy and radiotherapy and other therapies that are offered immediately to a cancer patient who has been diagnosed in an early stage, or in the later stage, Ayurveda also has certain treatments which can be given as an additional therapy along with these treatments. Something like catalyzing the main effects of those medications and also reducing the side-effects of those medications.

Other therapies that can help along with the main therapy would be something like meditation to generate the energy from the chakras, because there are chakras, which have connection to the various organs inside the body. There are six chakras, basically, according to the system of Yoga. There are particular hymns or mantras that can reenergize or bring harmony into those chakras again. When the patients who are suffering from such diseases are given the guidance to follow how to chant those mantras, that will continuously have an effect on those chakras and the harmony can be brought back. That is one type of treatment.

Another would be guided imagery. In this type of treatment, the patient is asked to imagine some foreign material or something like a devil or a demon inside the system - or in that particular place inflicted with cancer - and, take a breath, and in that breath, he or she sends an army, constituting his own body mechanism, defense mechanism, to that area to fight that demon and drive it out. Even this we have tried on some patients and it has contributed to a certain level of recovery. These are the other methods, which can be done.

Pranayama, that is rhythmic breathing, will also help to calm down the mind. There are many other methods - even music therapy will help in settling down the mind to bring tranquility.

According to the system of Ayurveda, mind and body are something like two sides of a coin. And whatever discomfort or disease is inflicted on the body will have an effect on the mind. And whatever discomfort or displeasure is there in the mind, the same will be inflicted or have an impact on the body also. So, the mind - with the will and determination - can control the body to a certain extent. And when these therapies are done indirectly, the mind will control the body in such a way, that the body develops the power to resist the disease.

When a patient comes to us with very low determination of mood, when he or she becomes aware that he or she has cancer, the first thing we have to do is offer reassurance that there are many methods to check the disease. So, the first thing is we have to give them reassurance. And, we have to give him or her all the facilities or advice that can give them strength to the body and mind. Also, we have to juggle proper treatment and programs for them and keep them busy, so that they should not be able to concentrate more and more on the disease. The first thing of importance is reassurance.

For some individuals who get cancer, it is something like - what do you call it - a total blow. It appears like a teacher, a hard taskmaster, at some level. So that all the abuse or stress or strain, which they have undergone all the years, requires them to learn to lead a more natural, a more regimented, a more determined and willful life. Because that will bring them good health for a longer duration or give them longevity.

There is a particular kind of harmony in the entire Universe. All the energies are flowing in a particular direction. According to the seasons, and the planets are moving in their orbits, and everything is controlled by a special force or energy which has to be in that particular state, in that particular time. And nature responds to it, and the physical and the mind also goes along with it. And when there is a disharmony, or something like it going against the current, this will result - not only in cancer - but that imbalance will cause diseases or a discomfort.

Something like when you're sailing in a river along with the current, it's easy. It's easy for you. You are going along with the current. But when you turn back, nature offers you a resistance. You have difficulty to go against the current. Similarly, nature has its own flow, the energy flow.

To have a complete idea of why a person becomes ill, that individual has to look back and into their life - regarding their diet, their activity, their food and their medications or stress, strain, their occupation, their daily routines. Each and every factor and how they've kept their mind, all these, they have to look and change it accordingly, one by one. Only then will they realize the difference. This is like straying out of the main highway path into a lane and later coming back to the main highway. That is the example given for the difference.

http://www.supremeayurcare.co.in/

Jeffrey Hollender

Co-Founder
Seventh Generation

Seventh Generation is a 21-year old company in Burlington, Vermont. We went into business to provide safer products for consumers, products that were safer for the planet as well as individuals who use them. We sell everything from cleaning products and laundry detergent and dish detergent to recycled tissue paper, baby diapers, wipes, even organic cotton tampons.

When we started the company, there was no such word as green products. Twenty-one years ago, people understood a little bit about water conservation and energy conservation, so we started by selling products that helped you use less water, energy efficient light bulbs, but there was no significant business around organic food. There was no such thing as organic clothing. We were very, very, very early - and we really catered to a pretty hard-core environmental community that was already aware of things like preserving forests, so they understood the benefit of recycled paper. The issues surrounding cleaning products were not understood at all. And it's hard to sell products to people when they don't understand why they need them or what problem they're solving. Thus, it was really a pioneering effort for the first decade we were in business.

Some of the issues we've tried to help people understand, with regard to cleaning products, are really most importantly health issues. It's important to understand that there is really no difference between a health issue and an environmental issue. The issues that affect our health adversely also affect the environment adversely. So systemically, this is all connected. But from a consumer perspective, certainly their health is a higher priority.

One issue that is very pronounced in the United States is indoor air pollution. The air in our homes is two to five times more polluted than the air outside of our homes. Why is that? Because we build homes with toxic chemicals and we bring toxic chemicals into our homes. That indoor air pollution has translated into incredible increases in things like asthma, allergies and chemical sensitivities.

We also look at things like cancer. Other than the reduction of cancer in the industrialized world because of people smoking less, virtually every other cancer is increasing. And the types of cancers that are increasing the quickest are cancers in children.

We have unleashed this gigantic chemical experiment on the population, which in the United States, is coming from the eighty thousand chemicals that are in production. Less than one percent of them have been thoroughly tested by independent, third parties for their safety. So we're the guinea pigs. Chemical companies make these chemicals, put them into products and sort of see what happens. And what's happening is not good.

We don't believe that you can put a little bit of a carcinogenic chemical in a product and tell consumers, "Well, there's such a little bit in there, it's not really going to matter." What happens is there's a cumulative effect. You get a little bit here, you get a little bit there, and all of a sudden you end up with cancer. Most of the business world operates on a principle that's sort of used in the legal system, that you're innocent until proven guilty. We don't think that that should apply to household products or personal care products.

At the end of the day, most consumers don't necessarily want to study thousands of chemicals and understand what is wrong with them or what dangers they hold. While we provide complete ingredient disclosure, so if you want to do the research you can, consumers trust us to select chemicals that are going to ensure their safety.

Unfortunately, consumers make this assumption that if a product is sold in a grocery store, someone has ensured that it's safe. Unfortunately, that's not the case. There is no independent authority that is approving and signing off on the cleaning products that end up in supermarket shelves. It's our responsibility as individuals to choose carefully. All you need to do is think about things like cigarettes. If we have a society where you can sell cigarettes, we have a society where you can sell cleaning products that could inflict equal damage. The standard to remove a consumer product or a chemical from distribution is so high and hard to meet that millions of dangerous products pass under that bar. And as parents, we learn to pay attention to the things we surround our children with. We want to protect them, because they can't protect themselves. We have to do that as adults. Unfortunately, we have to do the due diligence to ensure that we're buying safe products. And the easiest way the consumers do that is by choosing brands that they know do that for them.

Different parts of the world have different standards with regard to what chemicals are allowed to be used and what standards manufacturers must meet before they sell products to the public. In general, the European Union is much more strict than the United States. The United States is much more lax when it comes to toxic chemicals, when it comes to genetically modified ingredients. The U.S. really is the Wild West in a lot of respects when it comes to consumer products and chemicals. I think in thirty years we have barely removed ten chemicals from the market through regulation.

We know that there are thousands of chemicals that are suspected of being hormone disruptors, carcinogenic, chemicals that will adversely affect the ability of children to learn. We really have a huge health problem, whether it's allergies and asthma, which people are aware of, or attention deficit disorder. When you look at the cycle that society is in, you can see they don't regulate chemicals, thus consumer products have negative unintended consequences on the population, which then we treat by medication. The number of children that are using various types of medication to deal with health problems is a cycle that will only get worse and worse. You've got to remove the dangerous stuff, not treat people who then have adverse reactions to those chemicals.

While it's wonderful to have a great doctor who can help you make good choices and manage your care, I think Seventh Generation believes that responsibility starts with the individual. Whether it's very basic things, like diet and exercise, which are hugely important to our health, you can't get a pill to take care of your exercise needs. You have to take that responsibility. Healthcare in general is that way. It is much more effective, much more efficient, to be proactive than it is to get sick and go see the doctor and have them prescribe something for you. That's why in the U.S. healthcare costs are out of control, because we're treating the problem rather than avoiding causing the problem in the first place.

There is no way you can have a cost-effective healthcare system if people don't take some level of personal responsibility, which means that we have to educate people. We have to educate them so they know what choices to make. Today you read a magazine, you watch TV, there's a thousand people telling you a thousand different things to do. It's challenging and it's confusing. That goes back to the issue of trust. You need to have trusted sources, of not just products, but trusted sources of information.

The single most important change that needs to happen, that will do more to correct all of the problems and unintended consequences, is what I call full-cost accounting. So that if we buy something, or if a manufacturer sells something, the full costs are included. For example, soda, filled with sugar, is a reason why lots of people are obese or diabetic. If a soda company had to pay the cost of taking care of the people who were made ill by their product, soda might cost five or ten bucks apiece. Not so many people would be buying soda if it cost five or ten dollars. However, things like organic juice, which have health benefits, by comparison, would be cheap.

So, one of the challenges to overcome is we send all the wrong signals to consumers. Many of the things that are worse for us are cheapest and the things that are best for us are more expensive. That's the most important dynamic that has to change. By putting all of the costs into the products we buy, we will make it easier for consumers to make the right choices. So organic, natural, recycled, non-toxic products should cost less because they are more beneficial to society.

If a toxic product had to contribute to the cost of cancer

care, because it had a carcinogenic ingredient, it would be really expensive. But we have a system that lets business externalize those negative costs onto society. Because business doesn't have to take responsibility for those negative impacts, they can put all kinds of bad, terrible stuff in their products and not worry about the consequences. That dynamic is destructive. That dynamic is one of the flaws in the way we practice capitalism. It's not that I'm against capitalism, but the way we practice capitalism has a negative effect on the health, well-being - as well as the equity and justice - of our society.

I don't think that the large companies will make this transition on their own. They will make the transition because they want to mitigate some of the risks. Look at McDonald's. McDonald's has reduced the fat content and the calories of what they sell on their menu because they got worried about litigation, where families with obese children were going to come sue McDonald's for causing a bad health effect. That fear of litigation as a business expense will drive companies to do more of the right things.

But that's not enough. We need a combination of government regulation... Cap and trade, which is a mechanism to charge for CO_2 emissions, is one piece of full-cost accounting. But we need to do that with everything. We need to do that with sugar. We need to do that fat. We need to do that with all of the things that we sell. Businesses are making progress, but they're not making progress quickly enough. They won't make progress quickly enough on their own. We need a combination of NGO pressure and government regulation to create a playing field that is really level - where the bad stuff reflects that in its cost and the good stuff is priced accordingly.

One of the things that's important for consumers to do, and is really critical to begin to shift the dynamic, is to move beyond your consideration of an individual product and look at the whole company. One of the challenges that we face is that a company might make one good product and they might sell a hundred bad products. By your purchase of that good product from a bad company, you're supporting corporate practice that is having a very adverse effect on consumers. We've learned to become better about those individual product choices, but we haven't widened our lens to think about the company. We need to move from green products to supporting green companies, because today, one of the ways that many companies are mitigating their risk and trying to look good is by producing a few green products while they continue to do damage with the rest of their product portfolio. So one way to hold these large companies accountable is to not let them get by. Don't let them get by because they have a few green products. Push them to change their overall corporate practices and business purpose.

http://www.jeffreyhollender.com/

Aubrey Hampton

Founder
Aubrey Organics

I started working with my mother when I was about nine year's old making products. She was from La Costa, South of France. She was an herbalist and she made cosmetics. So I stood next to her side, learned all the different things that go into making a natural cosmetic. Of course, in those days there was no such thing as an organic cosmetic. That's changed now, but they were natural and she knew nothing about any kind of chemicals. So I only learned, or I did in fact learn, the right way. From there, I started my own company after I'd worked for other cosmetic companies - and carried on the tradition of my mother's company.

I guess it was a natural process for me to start the company. But probably what pointed it out more was my working for other cosmetic companies, becoming more and more cognizant of what went into cosmetics. When they called it natural, it wasn't really natural. Cosmetics were loaded with chemicals I'd never heard of. But of course, after I studied organic chemistry and got my PhD in organic chemistry, I did learn about all the different chemicals - what they represented, what they were used for, and I wanted to stay far away from them. It was really a conscious effort at looking at the world, looking at the environment, looking at people, looking how products went together - how they felt, how they worked. And that's what made it happen really. But I still have to say the background was there, it was put in place, because you can't go to a university and study cosmetic chemistry. It's something they don't give. You definitely can't study natural cosmetic chemistry. So, most of the chemists working in the cosmetic field come from other disciplines - and not necessarily how to put chemicals together that make cosmetics.

I personally know a lot about the chemicals that go into making cosmetics. And when I say chemicals, I'm referring to synthetic chemicals. I know a lot about them because I made it my business to know about them and to understand them - and understand all of the problems that are involved. But I was mainly interested in how hair and skin responded to natural products. What did it do, how did the skin feel? How did it work in a positive way for the people, and that's what I was after. I was after a product that does something, not that just says something, but a product that does something. That does something for the skin, does something for the hair, that is positive and makes you look great. That was my idea.

In the trade at the moment, you say, "What's out there?" It's the same thing that was always out there. There has not been a big change in something really being natural - or even the understanding of the word "natural" as it applies to a cosmetic. One of the early ideas was that the skin was like a canvas and everything lays on top of the skin. That was before they suddenly realized - because of hexachlorophene in chemical cosmetics that damaged and caused cancer - that it's not just a canvas, that it absorbs. And those absorptions go into the body and create a problem.

So the products that are out there on the shelves now, if you go into a supermarket or a drug store, they're the same products. Mainly what they do today, however, is they might put 'natural' on it.

I've always found that I like to write the ingredients on my products, because I am proud of what goes in them - and I want people to know what goes in them. So it was natural for me to always do that, even before it was a law in the '70s. I was doing it already. But you go on the shelf now, what do you find? You find the same old hair sprays with cold palmers and PVP. You find the same conditioners with guar propyltrimonium in it. So you find the same things, and what are these things? Well you have to learn about them. I did write about it in a book called <u>Natural and Organic Skin Care</u> where you can at least - it's like an encyclopedia where you can look it up. And you look it up and you find... Oh, now I know what sodium laureth sulfate is, now I know what guar propyltrimonium is, now I know what the erythrulose is, and now I know what methylparaben happens to be.

You would presume you can trust a cosmetic company, that they would not put something in their products that would harm you. I don't think they willingly put anything in their product that will harm you. It's what they do put in the product, for other reasons, that winds up harming you.

Probably the best thing to do is don't buy any product that has a chemical name in it that you don't understand. That would be the first step, just don't buy it. Don't use it. Why should you take a chance? There are perfectly good products out there that don't have the chemicals in them - don't do it.

In other words, don't let branding lead you astray. It is worth talking about branding. Every time we're talking about this, we're talking about advertising and branding.

"Our thing is good. Our thing is great. You're going to live and be young forever." That's what they do. But you've got to worry about what's in your cosmetics. You should become educated about it. I know a lot of people that buy my products are educated about it. That's probably why they buy my products that I manufacture, because they read the label and they say, "Oh, this looks good. This has none of those chemicals in it." That's what you have to do.

What do I say to a person that says, "I can't afford it?" All I can say to this person is that to do the best they can. Maybe if enough people are interested - and enough support comes from natural consumer organic committees and things - that will change. Maybe that will change. I am very optimistic that it will change.

So you spend a little bit more money for something that's natural - that's organic, that's good for you. Maybe that's a good idea. Maybe that's not a bad idea. Maybe it's expensive. Maybe it's worth the money. If you look at what doctor bills cost and what hospitalization happens - and the fact that you can get heart disease, you can get diabetes, you can get many diseases just from eating the wrong foods. It can happen. So, you want it as natural as you can, as organic as you can. That's what I call taking responsibility for your health. Who's going to do it for you? You have to do it for your children. But you have to do it for yourself, for your children, for your heirs, for your own body. You will feel better when you invest money in your health before you ever go to a doctor, before you ever go to a hospital, before you ever have a disease.

http://www.aubrey-organics.com/

Angela Stokes-Monarch

Raw Food Nutrition

To me, a large part of this journey is about taking responsibility for our own health and reclaiming our power. When I look around, I see so many people giving their power away to someone else, to other people. There's this sense that "I don't have the answers within me. I cannot take care of myself. I need a doctor. I need a psychiatrist. This person knows so much more about this than I do." That all feels very disempowering to me. I love to see people really take a step forward and say, "Actually, I came here in this body. Nobody knows more about this than I do. It can take care of itself if I fuel it with the right kind of fuel." So it's stepping away from the idea that everybody else out there has something else, that they know more about your body than you do. Stepping into that sense of responsibility, I think, is absolutely key. It's all about this idea of sovereignty. We can take care of ourselves.

Often when people hear about the idea of raw foods, the raw food lifestyle, they get freaked out. They think, "Oh my God, that must be so boring. What do you eat? You people just eat carrot sticks and celery sticks? I could never do that." We hear that so often. The thing with raw foods is that we've come to a point right now where you could literally create almost anything as a raw food dish from the cooked-food world. People are recreating and creating the most amazing, gourmet creations: pies and cakes and raw pizza, raw lasagna. All of those things might sound very bizarre if you've never had any exposure to them, but just get online or flip through a raw food recipe book and you'll see the kind of things that I'm speaking about. There are incredible resources out there these days for finding raw recipes. You can make it as gourmet as you like.

Some of the things that I enjoy myself; I might make a blended energy soup. So I'll put a load of vegetables in a blender together with some avocado and some lemon and garlic and blend it all up into a soup and I'll enjoy that with some flax crackers, let's say. So flax crackers are a way for raw foodists to replace breads. Giving up bread is usually the toughest thing for people, so flax crackers are a key part of that. There are many things that you can make like that - dehydrated foods will help you move away from all the cakes and cookies and breads and pastas and all those things that you might be used to.

Pasta is another thing. People often make zucchini pasta. There are little machines that you can use to make spiral shaped vegetables so you end up with these wonderful spaghetti-like zucchini. You can make your little tomato sauce or whatever you like and have that. There are lots of wonderful things you can create.

There's incredible raw food restaurants these days that you can take people to and show them that it doesn't have to be all apples and pears and boring. There's a huge amount of variety out there.

So when people are first starting out, there's a few things I love to share with them to maybe think about - to help them move into this in a way that feels gentle and loving and sustainable for them. Again, we don't want to just jump into being a hundred percent raw. For most people, that's not going to work out. One of the things is to start with fifty percent raw and take it from there. So what does that mean? I like to encourage people to ensure that fifty percent of the weight of the food going into your body, is raw food. So not the volume, but the weight of the food that's going into your body. That might mean for breakfast and lunch, every day, you eat totally raw. Then in the evening you eat something cooked or whatever you want to do. Maybe it means that at every meal you eat at least fifty percent raw. There're different ways of doing this. Maybe you make sure that all of your snacks are raw snacks. But just have that in your consciousness - that at least fifty percent of the weight of the food that's going into your body today is going to be raw food.

Start with the things that you know you like and just keep adding in more things. If you really don't like celery, don't eat celery. Don't think, "This is a raw food. I have to eat this." Forget it. You like blueberries, eat blueberries. It's all about taking little steps forward and replacing the highly toxic, refined food with things that you like, and are raw, and are coming straight from nature. So keep adding in things that you feel good about.

If you can have the intention to drink at least one green drink a day, that's going to be a wonderful healing aid for you as well. That might mean a green vegetable juice. It might mean a green smoothie, which is where you blend together fruit with leafy greens like spinach or lettuce or parsley or cilantro, all those kind of things. Blend those together in a blender with a little bit of water. You have an amazing drink that tastes good, which is great for beginners usually, or for children or reluctant spouses or whatever. It might even mean that you have a green powder. There're many different green powders you can buy out there in the market these days. Mix some of that up with a little bit of juice or water or whatever. Get the greens into you in whatever way you can.

Greens are what really help us to heal and feel balanced and alkalized. The greens are like the foundation for being happy and healthy. Eat salads. Eat the kind of green soups I was speaking about earlier, lots of vegetables blended together. Drink green drinks. If you can also manage to eat a little bit of seaweed everyday, that is also going to be a wonderful way of getting lots of minerals into your body. Now again, at the very beginning of the path, that might sound really odd and scary. "Eating seaweed every day? What is she talking about?" It's just something to keep in the back of your mind. It's something that over time maybe you'll feel more willing to incorporate.

The reason I feel it's absolutely key to get a lot of green foods into your body every day, is because greens have a massive amount of chlorophyll in them. Chlorophyll really, really helps us to heal. The chlorophyll structure is very similar to blood. There's actually only one atom different between chlorophyll and human blood. So when we take chlorophyll, or greens, into our body, it's almost, in a way, like having a blood transfusion. It's very cleansing for the body. It helps us to balance. Most people are in a state of a lot of acidity in their body, from the animal products and the highly refined foods, sugars, pastas, breads, all those kind of things. They're in a very acid state. When we take green foods into our body, it's very alkalizing. It helps the body to come into a state of homeostasis much more easily.

Along with that, depending on what the green foods are,

you'll probably find you've got quite a lot of minerals in there. Greens usually have a high percentage of amino acids as well, which are the blocks, the building blocks that go to protein.

The number-one question that raw foodists seem to be asked is, "Where do you get your protein from?" Greens are a huge part of that picture. When people eat very dense protein sources, like meat and dairy, it's very challenging for the body to break all of that food down. It's got to break it down into amino acids first and then use it to try and make some protein. It's a very energy-draining situation. Whereas, if you have the greens, you get all these live enzymatic amino acids coming straight into your body. Your body can just take that and go to work.

The classic thing that I always like to share with people when they ask me from where I get my protein: Where does a gorilla get its protein from? Where does an ox or a horse or a cow get its protein from? Look at those animals. They're like powerhouses. They're muscle-y, they're strong, they can run for miles. Where do they get their protein from? They're primarily eating greens. They're eating grass or leaves.

So work with what you've got, where you are. Read books. Keep inspired. Reach out to other people. Get support. Just take positive, little steps forward and don't overwhelm yourself.

http://www.rawreform.com/

Gerald Celente

Founder
Trends Institute

The first book I worked on in the mid-1980s was called
Natural Healing. My ex-wife was dying of Colitis. She was
down to 78 pounds. In the late 1970s we were living in
Chicago. We tried everything. We went to the University of
Chicago - a fellow from the University of Houston, seeking
out the best of what was being offered. We ended up in
Northwestern University and we went to see the head of
the gynecological department. They thought that she might
have some kind of other problem that was triggering the
colitis. I was a kid at the time and I was asking questions -
remember, this was the late 1970s. "Does diet make any
difference? What she's eating, would that help her at all?
How about vitamins?" I asked them about vitamins. People
were starting to talk about vitamins then. In those days,
they had one a day and that was it. The doctor got so
agitated he slammed down his pencil and he said, "I've
never been so grilled in all my life." He proceeded to throw
us out of the office.

We moved back East and we found a doctor, a
chiropractor, a chiropractic physician. His name was Jack
Soltanoff. He started teaching my wife about how to heal
herself. In those days chiropractic physicians, and probably
still today to some large degree, were the only ones that
were really dealing in alternative healing. You couldn't go to
your regular doctor and get any information about
acupuncture, about vitamin counseling, about diet,

nutrition. They didn't have a clue.

So we found this doctor up here. The first thing he did with her was to sign her up on a program. He started teaching us. Every Saturday we'd spend hours with him, learning about how to take care of our lives. The first thing with her was with diet. Colitis, we started thinking about it. I didn't know what colitis was. This doctor - by the way, the clown at Northwestern University, he wanted to put a bag in and give her a hysterectomy. She was thirty years old. So the first thing, I'll never forget, this doctor said, "A doctor is an educator and a teacher." So he started teaching us about taking care of ourselves.

The first thing he did was he put her on avocado and tomatoes in a blender. Think about how kind of soothing, but filled with nutrition and vitamins, that was. He said, "You can't eat empty, dead foods. They're not going to heal you." So it's part of the healing process. So as the food moved through the intestines, of course it was a smooth, nutritional food. It wasn't irritating the sores and the ulcers. It was one thing after another like this. Okra. Who the hell ever heard of okra? I'm a kid that grew up in the Bronx. I never heard of okra, that's a Southern food. But okra is mucous-y and filled with nutrition. So it was that kind of thing. It was one thing after another.

Heal yourself. Patient, heal yourself. That's one of the big trends that is going to happen. Heal yourself healthcare. If people haven't grown up enough to understand that their health is in their own hands, they're doomed. I can't believe how immature people are about this thing. They actually believe they're going to go to the doctor and the doctor is going to heal them. Yeah, in times of crisis you need that medicine, you need that emergency surgery. I live in the

Northeast. We have Lyme disease. It's a tic disease, tic-borne disease. I had it twice. Boy, you bet I went on heavy doses of antibiotics. I've seen the after-effects of people that didn't catch this thing in time. But that's only part of it. That's for the emergency.

A lot of diseases are stress-related. Where does stress build? Stress builds in the mind. You create your own stress, often. She came from a crazy, Italian family whose father was one of these...he would have been a great second for Mussolini. So yeah, she was uptight and she couldn't express herself. All those years of living in fear, you get tightened up. So it was a whole process. It's not one-dimensional.

She became a martial artist. She went from a skinny, little dying girl to a top-flight martial artist in close combat. She's my ex now. I haven't seen her in a number of years. When she left she was in great shape.

People are living, they're partially conscious basically, in the sense that they're running to work, their lives are filled with so many different things. They're not taking time to study and learn about what's going on. What they're hearing are bits of propaganda, basically, from the major media. So they think what they're hearing - all of a sudden they become instant experts and put a whole analysis together and move forward on what they hear.

In the States we have an obesity problem. They're estimating that in the next seven years, over forty percent of the adults are going to be obese in the States, thirty percent of the children. What are they doing now? The drug companies push out this study that just came out yesterday. The "New York Times," the paper of record, promoted "Test your children for cholesterol problems now. Then put them on statins, on cholesterol-lowering drugs." Hey, how about telling your kid to stop eating a lot of crap? Maybe that'll help. People are too damn lazy to take care of their own lives. Yeah, stop going to McDonald's and Burger King and every other fast food joint. Stop drinking all this soda, Red Bull, phosphorescent slurpies, Mars Bars and maybe you'll be okay. So I mean, it's insanity!

It's difficult. I mean, every day I get on the scale. I love eating. I'm Italian. I love food. I've been fifteen pounds heavier than I am. I'm a small guy. It's tough to lose weight. Every winter I have to lose weight, every summer, because I put on so many pounds. It's work. But it's respect of yourself. That's all it comes down to. It's about you. The healthier you are, the healthier the people around you are going to be: physically, emotionally, spiritually. They're going to be healthier. So it's up to you to really take control. It's about what you want in your life.

For me, when I have my last breaths, I want to know I was true to myself, that I lived up to the standards that I set for myself. So really, staying in good shape and staying in good health is about really respecting yourself. End of story.

A lot of people don't have healthcare. They're going to have to take care of themselves. There are more educated people that realize that every drug that they take has a side effect, like death, and they don't want to take these drugs. So you're going to have a combination of two things. People are going to have to go on an economic slim-fast and a health slim-fast. It's going to be forced upon them. The more intelligent people will understand that the higher the quality of food that goes into you, the higher the quality of your health, often.

This Dr. Soltanoff, he used to follow this food-combining thing, about not mixing proteins and starches and that type of thing, which I happen to agree with. If you're going to eat fruit, that's a meal. Fruit is a meal. It's a whole meal. It's not fruit after the meal, it's not fruit with - it's the meal. But whatever your thing is, the thing is, learning about food, learning about the highest qualities, looking at food as nutrition...people will spend how much for a gallon of petrol? How about buying some high-quality food and putting it in there, rather than shoving crap down your mouth?

I believe the great pandemic is going to be cancer, brain cancer, from all these cellular waves pounding into the brain. One study after another is showing the possible damages. They keep pushing it under the rug. Then they're wiring their kids up. The studies are coming out showing - French studies, Danish studies, Swedish studies, Israeli studies, English studies - the thinner the brain shield on the kid, the deeper the waves go in. I think there's going to be a pandemic, worldwide, particularly in the developing nations as well, because they're on only cells. They have these microwaves blasting in. You don't think it's going to hurt? Great, keep doing it. I don't own a cell phone.

People have to start taking responsibility for their lives. So what are you going to do? Grow up. Take life into your own hands. The Internet makes it more and more possible and feasible to seek out the best of what's available. It's there in front of everybody.

http://www.trendsresearch.com

Max Harrison

Aboriginal Healer
Australia

My name is Max Harrison, and I've been working with "bush stuff" for as far as I can remember. I've been taught by some of the elders that have given me some information on plants and whatever they know, to do healing. A lot of my stuff was handed down by some, whom I call masters - not teachers - but masters. They had the legacies of around eighty thousand years of knowledge that they sort of dealt with. So, I was good enough for them to pass that information on to me. I felt privileged in the 40s and 50s to be able to sit with some of the elders - to learn a bit about the environment and what it produces.

You never approach the elders. They always approach you, or pick you out, and they watch your discipline to see how you react to what you're being told - how you react around family: the aunties and uncles, grans and pops. The masters, the elders, would sit down and they would talk about you. They'd say, "This kid here is asking why and what for - and so he looks to be someone we can take and do some teaching with."

When I was down the coast, I started to do a bit of that and practice some of the knowledge that was handed down to me. That was important. I still had to get permission from the elders. I don't mean the living elders, the spiritual elders. Those old people would still somehow consult me and give me a message - of what to give that fellow or this one here, what to do with them.

I deal a lot with spirit, and that's where I get a lot of my knowledge. I get it as well from the living elders and masters.

Plants, herbs, water, winds, areas. It's not all just plants, or it's not all just your herbs and your other stuff. It's about water also, and it's the localities, which is very important in how you can take people out and sit with them and talk about their sicknesses. Sounds are another thing that I was told to use - sounds and the feeling of energies.

When you talk to somebody about their illness you can - because what they're telling you is a result of a cause or something that's happened to them, or something that they ate or something that they're worried about - start to look at that and you start to say, "Hang on." This person has gone beyond the physical part now of needing help. This person needs to be first talked with and nurtured in an inner sense - so they can start to see where their sickness is coming from. That's a very important part of looking with their voice. It's like when you walk into the bush you look at the language of the land, you don't listen. But you look at the language of the land, and the land can tell you a lot of things - of what is and what it can generate and what it can offer you. And you start to notice those things, and you can start to communicate with that by understanding.

It's just like looking at an old tree. An old tree looks to be so disease-ridden. Somebody will come along and say it could be two or three hundred years old. And that old tree that's standing there - some people would see it's ready to be cut down - it will fall down on someone, or it will fall down on somebody's property. Or, it may come down because people are only looking at the financial part. You see, they're not even looking at the healing capacity of that old tree. Then I start to look at all the different aspects - from the root to the bark to the sap to the leaves to the limbs to the leaves to the blossoms of that particular tree. Then you know, okay, there is a healing substance that can do some human good, because that's the land talking to you. That's the land speaking the language of silence, the beautiful language of silence that we as a human can't understand - or don't understand or don't want to understand. I start to look at that beautiful healing capacity that the old tree has got.

One of the reasons people are getting cancer, I'd say, is wrong foods. Worry is another thing. Because sometimes, when you worry about something, you get a headache. What was demonstrated to me once by the masters, they showed me that formula - your two brains - your coordinating brain and your thinking brain. I learned that once these things start to happen, and you worry about it, and the messages that go through your body - your skin starts to either crawl or jump. And so does your nervous system. All these things happen like that, just by worrying. So, if you just keep worrying, every fiber in your body can get manipulated and cracked up - that's what the masters taught me.

Sometimes when people have got cancer, and they find out they have cancer, it's pretty well advanced within most of them. Of course, the panic button is pushed and they want to try to get healed. They want to get healed, and boy, you know, they're clutching at straws - and so it's so hard for them. The mind just keeps going back and feeding the sickness.

Having the "lore" of acceptance of what sickness they have - if they can hold on to that law of acceptance and then start looking for answers - because all of your body tells every other little bit of you inside. So every time you have that law of acceptance, you can deal with whatever problem you got. To not intensify the spreading of the disease. You can hold that back and go on. Just find the most suitable herbs and medicine and live your daily life. That's important.

So, that's where your law of acceptance is the best thing. So, you found out now that you have this sickness, so what can you do about it? You start working with your positive thoughts so you can start trying to find a healing method - or try to find a healing medicine. And if you keep going like that, something will come through for you. You can put the disease into remission yourself, because if you're worried, then it flares up everything. "Healing thyself" is such an important thing, "heal thyself."

There's a word there that the doctor will say. You have an "incurable" disease. And what does that do? It puts it back into that irrational mind again. So "incurable" disease, you leave it out of your vocabulary. That's a negative thing that you're taking on board. We got to learn to start to kick out the negative and just hold the positives, and then we can start working on self. Or, if you hurt yourself and you're in a lot of pain, shift the pain. Shift the pain. These things are so important to learn about self - and do something about self and not just rely on the drugs and that. There's a lot you can do with your mind. You can change things, you can start moving pain, you can start doing a lot of things with your mind to start to heal yourself.

So where's your lore of acceptance? It's gone out the window, it's gone out of your persona. You never, ever do these kinds of things. You hold it, you hold that lore. That l-o-r-e is the most important of acceptance, and "Yes, I'm healing, I'm going to heal, and I'll stay healed" and they go into remission.

My first thing was with an old mate. He was from the North Coast and a beautiful man. I took him through alcohol recovery, and it was so wonderful to see him go through that and come out the other end. I went back home to the far South Coast. Someone told me, "You're old brother Bob's in hospital, and he's got cancer." I said, "Oh my goodness," and I went to see him. He was in the hospital laying up, and I walked in and he said, "Isn't it funny you helped me get rid of one disease and that is alcoholism? Now, I've beat that one, and that's the one I wanted to beat. "Now what comes? Now, what I've found out is, I've got cancer." I said to him in a joking way - I didn't want it to be blame, but I did it in a funny way - I said, "You know you gave up booze, but you kept on bloody smoking, you clown." I said it like that, and he said, "Oh yeah, I was still puffing on the old fags."

Then he shut up and he looked at me and said, "How you brought me through alcoholism, I'm going to try now to go through this - what I got here in the lungs and that." I said, "Okay, do you want me around?" He said, "You taught me one thing about self-healing. You taught me about self-healing." I said, "Tell me, how long did they give you, brother?" He said, "A few weeks," and I looked at him and said: "For someone who's going to kick the bucket in three weeks, you're pretty laid back about it." He said, "About what?"

You see what he had done there? He said, "About what?" Of course, then I shut up also. I said, "About why

154

you're laying in the bloody hospital." He said, "I won't be here too long." He said it like that. "I won't be here too long." So, I hugged him for a while and I said, "If you want me, get a hold of me, get someone to get in touch with me and I'll come and sit with you."

And it wasn't until about eighteen months later, I wonder how Bob is? I rang up the North Coast to see where he was, and I said, "Is old Bob around?" - "Oh yeah, he's down there fishing, down on the rocks fishing." Then the old guy dies in a car accident. He died in a car accident three years later. That was him and I left him. I didn't have to be there with him. I just left him the legacy of what to do and he took it. The same as he'd done with the booze. This is how people can heal, self-healing.

When you look at the doctors, God bless them, some of them try. They're handy to have there in emergencies. I would never condemn a doctor, but sometimes - when it comes to taking out a bit of that cancer, opening you up - I believe and I know that causes more damage than anything. Because what I keep looking at is that old grandfather tree and how damaged he was, and how he's still standing there after about two or three hundred years old and still as strong as ever. He's getting all this stuff from the land to keep him standing strong.

Once they stay in "sorry time," their spirits are low and that spirit's got to recover, that spirit's got to come back. You'll hear people talking about fighting the spirit. They don't want to just talk about it, they have to practice it. Practice what you preach is such an important thing in your healing.

Dan Ariely, Ph.D.

Placebo Effect

My name is Daniel Ariely and I'm the James B. Duke Professor of Behavioral Economics at Duke University. I also have an appointment in the Business School in Cognitive Neuroscience, which is a separate department in the economics department. I do research on irrationality.

I look at all kinds of economic decisions made - but not necessarily assuming they're irrational. I do different experiments to figure out how people actually behave, and then I try to think about what are the consequences of this thing for the market, for the economy, for society?

There are a lot of curious things about being in the hospital, but one of the interesting things was as a burn patient; I would keep very close track as to how much pain medication a physician would allocate to me every day. There was a description of how many dosages, how many milliliters of different painkillers we could get. And I would track how much I'm getting and how much do I have, and I would try to kind of reason and ration myself. But in the process, I also tracked other people - what were they having, how were they rationing it and so on. Of course nobody was in the room with me - I was in the burn department and it's important to keep everybody separate for reason of infection - but I would track what other people were getting. And sometimes at night, I would hear some patients scream from pain and the nurses would come and give them their medication. And I would ask how often are you giving them, as they'd passed their limit.

Or, I'd ask what's going on or maybe could I get some more? And often, they would tell me that they just give them placebos - saline, water with a little bit of salt - and I was shocked that they were giving it to them. But even more surprising was the fact that after they would get the saline, they would fall asleep. And you'd say, how is this possible? Now, I don't know if they gave it to me ever or not. Of course if they told me, it would never have worked.

It's really incredible. It's one thing to believe in placebos and read the papers about it. It's a completely different thing to see somebody who is screaming for pain get an injection, which is nothing but salt water, and getting them to feel all of a sudden much, much better. It's really an incredible thing.

I think that's the body's inherent ability to heal itself, so when you expect a painkiller, your body excretes opioids. It basically secretes a substance very much like morphine. Regrettably, when you're in pain, you can't close your eyes and say, "God, can I get some pain killers?" Or, you can't say, "Brain, can I please get some pain killer?" It's something we do, but we don't have volitional control over it.

When we get an injection, when we pop a pill, when we do something, we trust somebody. And all of a sudden, our body in preparation for that effect is producing the effect. This is the best example of the self-fulfilling prophecy, where you believe in something and this actually gets your body to behave in a way that makes it real. That's the magic, right? You expect the pain reduction, you're getting something like a pill or injection, and your body creates the pain reduction you expect it to get - even if the pill is nothing. Now, in that sense, placebo is real. It's real because it has a real physiology. It just doesn't have to be about the injection or the pill; it's about moderating and changing our own physiology as a consequence of outside intervention. That's the magic in placebos. That's basically what sustained medicine for a very long time. It's, even now, a big part of modern medicine.

Placebo is not bad. Placebo is wonderful. We have an unbelievable immune system. If we understood how our immune system worked, we would kill a lot of cancerous cells. We would overcome a lot of diseases. The body is really wonderful. Placebo is a way to get the body to work better, to harness the power of our own abilities for a better cause.

My sister-in-law is a physician and she started practicing in India. She said that in India about two thirds of the patients would start to feel better the moment they would see her. They would come into the room and they would already feel confident, good about it almost immediately.

She said when she started practicing in the U.S., she gets much less of that. It's not because we are healthier as a nation. I think it's because we trust our physicians less. So in India, she had two functions. She was a trusted source - maybe a visual placebo - that the moment people saw her, they felt better and she was also practicing medicine. In the U.S., her placebo effect is lower and therefore she is less effective.

Now, will there be time when we don't need physicians? No, I don't think so. I think physicians are incredibly important. Medical science is incredibly complex. In fact, it is so complex that most physicians don't understand it very well. There are these incredible abilities of our bodies, but we do want to get some advances from external influences.

And how do you get both of them? You have to get physicians to help you - and I think their role will only become stronger as we develop technology, more complex drugs, more specific ideas as to what drugs fit which people and so on. Their role will just increase.

It turns out the desire for patients to come out with something in their hands is also something very common in India. It's not just in the U.S. You can think about it: For a real placebo effect to happen, you want to take something. You want to feel that you've done something that then releases the power of placebos. There are a lot of rural practitioners in India who give people one dosage of antibiotics, or they give them half an hour of an IV, or give them small things that get people to feel better.

The number of people who leave a physician without a prescription is very close to zero. Even for viruses, people give antibiotics. The doctors know it's not going to work. But of course, what are they going to do? They want to make the patient happy and the patient is going to take the pill and feel better. It's kind of a terrible cycle because, all of a sudden, we're creating more bacterial resistance to antibiotics; we're not helping the health of people and so on. It would be much better if the physician could actually prescribe placebos that don't have the negative side effects of antibiotics.

We developed this fantastic drug called Valedone RX that took many, many hours to come up with the name. That was it, it was just a name, there was nothing else in it. And basically we tested how Valedone RX worked as a pain medication. So we bought people to the lab and we connected them to a machine that would give them a set of electrical shocks.

But before we would connect them to a machine, we wanted to make them feel like they were in a doctor's office. So we had someone wearing a white lab coat, with a stethoscope. We asked them questions about their health, their family health and so on. We measured their heart rate, their blood pressure. Then we connected them to this machine, and we gave them a set of electrical shocks. And for each, we basically asked how painful was this on a scale of zero to a hundred, using a visual analog scale. Not painful to the most pain they could imagine. They would say this, this, this. Shock - this level, shock, this level - and so on.

Then when they finished going through a whole set of shocks, we gave them a brochure about Valedone RX and then we gave them the pill. It was a beautiful red pill, which turned out to be Vitamin C, but they didn't know it. And then we gave them fifteen minutes to read old "Newsweek" and "Time" magazines - to really make them feel as if they were in a doctor's office. Then, we connected them again to the machine and gave them a second set of electrical shocks. And then, we compared how they reacted to the first set of shocks with the second set of shocks. So there was the first set of shocks, a pill, then a second set of shocks. Will they feel less pain in the second set than the first one? And the answer is absolutely yes.

That's basically the placebo effect. The moment you take something, you feel less pain on the second set. But what we also did was give different people different brochures about Valedone RX. Some people were told it was an expensive pill; some people were told it was a cheap pill. Some people were told that it was made in China; some people were told it was made in the U.S. So we had four

160

conditions in total. Cheap in China, expensive in China, cheap in the U.S., expensive in the U.S. Basically, what we saw was that the expensive Valedone worked much better than the cheap Valedone. The level of pain decrease between the first set and the second set was much bigger for the people who got the expensive pill - compared to the people who got the cheap pill.

We also saw that the Chinese medication, surprisingly to us, did slightly better than the American medication - but it only did better for the people from South Asian origin. So it wasn't for Caucasian people. For Caucasian, there was no difference. But for the people with South Asian origins, the Chinese medications actually did slightly better. You can think that maybe it was because they were thinking about Chinese medication - that it invoked some good healing power, and so on, so it did slightly better.

When we asked people what they thought of Valedone RX, people loved it; they thought it was a fantastic pill. Imagine that you went through this experiment, you experienced some pain, got a pill and you experienced the same pain to a much lower degree. You would say, "Where can I get this wonder pill?" And they were really shocked to figure out that it was just placebo - but they were also very amused and interested at the idea, because this is exactly what happened to people in the hospital. Imagine you could go through this experience - when you don't know when at some point someone will give you a placebo - and say that this pain reduction you just felt was nothing but the creation of your own mind. There was nothing in the pill itself. It's really an incredible thought.

The power of placebo basically comes from two aspects, both through associations. The moment you expect something to be good, it's better because you expect it to be good. It's also due to classical conditioning. You must remember this thing from experiments of Pavlov, right? There was a dog, there was meat, there was a bell. There was bell, meat, salivation, bell, meat, salivation and so on and so forth - until at some point, the salivation moved in time to be closer to the bell, and the food was not needed. So there was bell, salivation. That's one of the ways that placebo works. You pop a pill, you take an injection, you think something is happening - and in the expectation of this reality, your body is preparing for that new future. There's a consequence creating that. Imagine if we just ordered pizza and the doorbell is ringing. We both know the pizza is coming, like the dog - and as a consequence, your juices in your stomach will start flowing, preparing yourself for the effect of eating pizza. Changing the physiology of your body is nothing more than expectations.

The same thing happens with all kinds of placebos. You expect something to happen, your body is preparing for the future - and the process of preparing for that future is changing the physiology of ourselves into something else.

It's hard to close your eyes and say, "Please, please, can I get some pain relief from you, mind?" It's very hard. If you think about placebo, if you think about classical conditioning, Pavlov's dogs could not start salivating by making themselves salivate. You cannot, to a large degree, imagine pizza and start salivating. You really need the door, the external stimulus to do it. You know, maybe with practice we could do it. Maybe Yogi masters can have better control of their minds. But for most of us, it's very, very hard - and that's why we need to take different things to get our body to react in the way that we expect.

The more optimistic part about placebo is to basically see how much your own body is doing and how can you get it to do more. For each person, it might be a different approach. If you think that relaxation works - maybe there's no particular science that shows that relaxation works for something - but if you think it's working, it might actually work for you. Anything that increases people's trust and expectations could actually have a big effect. We are an active participant in the healing process. We're not the mechanical creature of having an input from the medicine. It has a very fixed effect. In fact, our own body interacts with the medications in all kinds of ways. It depends on our experience, expectations, hopes and so on. Therefore, the final effect is a compound of those things.

What's happening in the immune system in this modern world? One thing we know for sure is that stress has a huge impact on the immune system. There are different types of stress, and different types of stress have different effects on different parts of the immune system. But overall, stress is incredibly bad for the immune system.

The other thing we know is that we now live longer. Because we live longer, we have more chances to get different diseases. So cancer, as an example, every one of us gets multiple episodes of cancers in our lifetime. In most cases, our immune system is able to handle it and it goes away. In some cases, it does not. It's a game, like going to Las Vegas. You're playing the odds and sometimes it fails. If you live ten years, the chances of getting cancer are very low. If you live eighty years, it gets higher. If your immune system is weaker, because of stress, then chances are that you will be even more likely to get cancer.

For example, they take rats and they give them stress in

the following way: they give them electrical shocks at unpredictable times. So imagine you have rats, they get electrical shocks and you have other rats that get a signal beforehand that a shock is coming - and then they get a shock. It would be a bell. So some rats just get shocks at unexpected times and other rats get a hint in front of it that there is a shock coming. It turns out that the first set of rats, the ones that don't get the signal, are much more likely to get cancer. That's stress, right? Something is coming at them. All kinds of things are happening to them. They don't know where they're coming from. Because of that, their immune system is much reduced and the chances of getting all kinds of diseases are elevated.

There used to be a particular operation people did for heart attacks. Physicians would basically cut people open and narrow some of the blood vessels. They did it for many, many years until somebody decided to do a placebo study and do a sham operation - and to simply cut people open, go into the heart and do nothing. Turns out these people felt the same relief as the other people.

Now again, one perception is to say these are terrible operations. The second thing is to say these are wonderful placebos. It's incredible that you can do something without cutting - and just getting people's expectations high can actually have some efficacy.

http://www.danariely.com/

Tony Samara

Spiritual Teacher
Author

Why is there an increase in the cancer rate, especially in the West? It's increasing everywhere. One obvious reason - it's not obvious maybe to everyone - but, one obvious reason is that today we live in a world that's totally different and changing more rapidly than fifty years ago, a hundred years ago, two hundred years ago and how primitive people lived. I call them primitive, meaning that they lived more in harmony with nature. The major reason I see is that we're changing the whole structure of what supports life, and that is nature. We do this by creating more pollution, by creating more radiation; by creating more aspects of civilization that interfere with our natural rhythm. This natural rhythm then gets depleted and doesn't have time to reinforce itself so that the healing can happen more easily.

For example, you could go to what the Swiss call sanitariums, places of healing such as in the mountains or in a forest - where people could breathe fresh air and people could just feel the elements work on their physical well-being. It's not so easy today, for most people, because they don't live in those circumstances. They live in cities or towns or in places where there is industry, and all this affects modern human beings. And perhaps it explains why we as modern human beings suffer from the cancer rates that are increasing. And, this involves specific cancers that are today very common, which were not common at all in the primitive world. This is one major reason.

Also, food, I feel, is a very important reason. The food that we eat is modern food. It lacks the vitality of coming straight from nature. It's processed. The way it's processed and the chemicals that are added to this processing of food - and the way it's cooked and the way it's eaten even, like fast food - all affect this vital system in our body. So of course, we get depleted in our healing system, which is very, very strong. It still works, but at times where there is a crisis or where there is a situation where the healing loses its path, then the cancer takes over in the body. It becomes much more dominant than it should be.

When I say this, it's just to highlight that cancer isn't something that happens overnight. It's a whole process. We all have a little bit of cancer in our body, but it goes crazy, so to speak, becomes a real cancerous growth when that vital system loses it's power. And the reason it loses its power, or one of the big reasons, is because of pollution and because of the way we eat. Another big reason is because of the state of affairs that we are living in the modern world. This can be explained in the culture that we live in, which is a culture, I believe, a culture, a beautiful culture, but that has a lot of fear and a lot of limitations. This stops people from really expressing who they are, and from being free in who they are.

Stress can be good, if it helps people move in a certain way. But stress that becomes depleting, because it has fear, has a weight to it, creates this mental anguish. But that, I feel, is one of the reasons why cancer is increasing. So even if we're not aware of it, a lot of our culture becomes incorporated in who we are, in our personality, and of course this creates an unconscious stress. And we only become aware of it when we step out of that picture. So when people get cancer, very often they realize - and this is part of the growth - that life has much more, shows much more of itself than is ever possible before the cancer. Because you're forced in a way to face aspects of yourself that before were unconscious, were not seen, or were mundane to your everyday existence. But then these aspects become very important for you to look at because you realize that it's part of the bigger picture, creating this unease in the body, this disease in the body.

Do people have the capacity to heal themselves? It's an interesting question, because if one says no - in the way of some type of action, which is, for example, and I'm not criticizing doctors here - through lack of choices common in some of the modern medicine today where the doctor takes the power away by saying you are sick and this medicine may help - then it creates a distrust in the lack of healing capacity that the body has. The body actually has this healing capacity that is so unlimited, so strong, that we only realize it when we believe that it is possible. We can actually facilitate that healing in ourselves, through the belief system or through working energetically and mentally and emotionally with what that means.

Everyone has the capacity to heal their sickness, many things. But many people have forgotten how or they've given that authority to do so to a situation that's external to themselves. So given either to the doctor or to a situation that may be a process - a dynamic that is strong outside of themselves. For example, it might be a situation that makes them angry and they become addicted to a certain pattern or state of being involving that situation. So an alcoholic, for example, can create this by stopping to be an addict in the sense of what society sees as an addict - drinking too much alcohol. But, the process that created that addiction in the first place is still there on the outside - and of course on the inside. The outside being the dynamics that created this problem in the first place. If that is not resolved, then that creates the sickness. Because the person doesn't see that situation is taking away their power to actually heal what is going on through their belief system and their own capacity to heal their body.

For me, the first step - I suppose this is part of the question, the first step to take when you get cancer, is to acknowledge what that means, totally. And this is what people don't do. Most people react to it from either their fear, which is socialization, or they react to in a way that completely stops the whole process from going further - it stops it at that point.

Every person who is sick, I believe has the answer inside, must know that part of the sickness is also part of the cure. But the cure is only part of the sickness to you individually, so it cannot be so specific as saying, "This is the right way to follow, and this is step number one, this is step number two." This is why it's complicated to address very clearly, because everyone is so different.

So, to generalize and to make it more understandable for someone who has cancer, it's acknowledging what this really means. The acknowledging is not just in a physical sense, you know, saying you have cancer, but in an emotional and a mental sense, and an energetic sense - maybe some people say spiritual sense. How does it really fit in now, in this moment, to your life? And taking time - that's what people forget to do - to take time. Not just to panic and rush and try to find a solution, but to take time and sit, or stand or whatever, enjoy. It's difficult to enjoy when you have this problem, but to enjoy the space that is created in that moment, with this new dynamic that's thrown in. And then we open up a gateway to seeing something that is totally different in relationship to the so-called disease.

The thing is that disease is not an external thing. And so, it's not about accepting something that is foreign to you. It's about accepting a part of yourself. And I think that when people realize that cancer is a part of them, and it's not something that's come to punish them, or something horrible that's happening to them, and all the ideas that come out of limited thinking - which comes from socialization, which comes from fear - then you open a completely different picture of what disease means. So then you can approach it, not just by owning up, but by loving and embracing this part of yourself in a different way. And that allows for something to speak to you from deep inside, from your heart, from the inner core of your wisdom. And that helps you to really see what steps you need to take because then it comes from a different dimension of yourself. It doesn't come from a reaction or fear or reaction of "My gosh, what's happening to my body?" - but comes rather from a more holistic background, deep from inside of yourself. And then, you trust yourself and you empower yourself in the process to allow you to choose what is really correct, to work with this situation.

And no one can tell you. You know in the end. It's your own intuition that will really speak as to what is best to do. Animals do this all the time. This is why they have less cancer. They have a more direct line of communication to their instincts and to their core than human beings. Human beings have had to adapt to modern society. So they have to go through many phases, which I call a process, before they can come directly to that answer.

So if you look at the present moment, then you can see the factors that are playing into this moment, into your life, into your emotional life, into your physical life, into your mental life, that are creating disharmony. This is very easy to look at, once you begin to actually look at it. Normally life is so busy that we don't have time to look at it, but when you have cancer, then your priorities change and you begin to say, "Okay, gosh, I didn't realize that this actually disturbed me so much." When you realize, then you can address it immediately and begin to change it. So you can begin to change, for example, work. If you're not happy in work - and you've just been working because you have responsibilities - and you see you have a situation that forces you to be in that working environment. Now that you have cancer you realize, hopefully, you realize, "I don't need to put myself in that situation anymore. I can go beyond it." Maybe cancer helps you in that respect.

So you address all the specifics that create disharmony in your life. This is not so much about going back and finding out, "Gosh, when I was ten this happened and then all of a sudden that may have created anger in my feelings." It's not so important, because what is more important is how you put it into action now. What does that mean to you as a person now - in this present moment - in relationship to a partner? In relationship to your friends? In relationship to your work, in relationship to food, in relationship to the environment that you're living in, in relationship to yourself? How you treat yourself, and what you do and how you think about yourself energetically, emotionally, matter. All this is in the present moment. There is no need to go back too far, unless there is a real major trauma, which isn't always the case if you have cancer. It doesn't mean if you have cancer, you've had a very traumatic history. It can mean that, but it's not always the case.

I think a mental attitude - and the time it takes to create that mental attitude - is one thing that's missing in modern medicine. The word cancer evokes so many images in people's mind. It's very difficult to be positive with those images. If the doctor says, "Sorry. I'm afraid to tell you. I'm really sorry that you have cancer and you have six months to live." Or, "It's likely that you'll get sicker two years from now." However they put it. It's very difficult to be positive, to leave the room, because it's about you. And you're dealing with a reality that isn't a program on the television or someone else that you're hearing about. It's you. You react. It's difficult not to react.

The attitude of being positive - it's not so much that you say, "Ha, ha, this doesn't mean anything to me and I'm fine" - that can be a way of escaping from the reality of what it means to you. It's more about detaching and finding a space that is free from getting so connected to that negative aspect. That detachment isn't a sense of joy all the time. It can be a sense of seriousness. You could, through that sense of seriousness, realize what it means to be alive and appreciate aspects such as stillness, such as peace, such as yourself, that become forgotten in life.

And some people say, "The cancer has been the best thing in my life, because it's made me see and live life in a way that I couldn't have done prior to the cancer." And, you know when you can see that, of course, that sets in motion a whole healing system - the vital system is acknowledged and is in more harmony with itself. So, of course, that attitude - when it comes from deep inside - it's not just a superficial attitude. It brings that space into more action. So that space then brings other actions, other ways of doing things, that heal the person in unexplained ways.

Everyone has that potential to create a miracle for themselves. It's much more than going to a doctor, and it's much more than finding a remedy. It's about something that is a whole process. Once that process is set in motion, it's a beautiful process. Actually, sometimes people who have cancer help give that beauty to other people in the family, helping them acknowledge that beauty which they wouldn't have seen - because the process is not about an individual. The process is about family, community and society. So often through cancer, many people see things that normally would have been impossible. It's such a beautiful thing.

I think this is the other part of what is forgotten - creating a space where there is joy, where there is peace, where there is harmony, not just with oneself but with everything that is around. Once this happens, it's an amazing thing. So often, the person then will say, "Wow, I can just do this. I don't have to be in this situation. I can just do this." But it comes from a space of experience. It's not like someone saying you have to do this to achieve that. The person realizes that for himself. This frees him or her from the stress that created the cancer in the first place. It could be, for example, a situation of anger, that they're angry deep inside and they don't know it. Then they realize that they don't have to be angry, that anger is a level of communication that's limited - and that you can communicate more deeply to a person than just being angry. That communication in itself is such a gift. It's a gift for all humanity. When you partake in that gift, you invite other people to communicate to you, so you realize you're not alone, with no reason to be angry. Then you are somehow participating in the healing more than the healer. You're actually doing something specific, if it's you who is creating the space.

For some people, maybe they need to go through the medical system. However, this choice doesn't have to be that they say no to seeing the disease as a beautiful gift. They can go through the medical system and encompass many other aspects of the disease in a more holistic way. Or, some other people may choose to go through an alternative route, whatever that is. Again, that doesn't mean you have to focus just on that. If you take into account more the whole perspective of things, then I think the healing happens on a much deeper level - so that the cancer doesn't come back. And, you can understand what the cancer really means to you - so that you do not fear if it will come back as a negative aspect that you have to push away.

One thing is to remember is that cancer requires negative to flourish on. When I say negative, in the physical sense, negative is pollution. So, if you are living in a polluted environment - or if you have channels where you have pollution coming into your body - then of course, if you have cancer, the body is saying, "Please, I don't want any more. Please make sure that whatever is coming in is supporting the vital energy rather than depleting the vital energy."

So this is done basically through food. There are so many books that explain how to do this. But more importantly, we need to know illness can also come through the air that we breathe. I think one of the major reasons why people get sick is because of pollution, the air that we breathe. The pollution that we breathe into our bodies minimizes the amount of oxygen that comes into the physical organism - into the cells of the body. And, this is one thing that, of course, creates physical disease that people forget about. We get used to living in a city, breathing in the fumes, breathing in something besides fresh air. This is one thing, if you have cancer, maybe to look at.

Now if you have cancer, why not go to a place where you can breathe in fresh air? Practice certain meditations that help to breathe in more deeply. Work on elements in yourself that help to limit the negative perspective of breath. That means if you're angry, to work on joy, to work on happiness. So the breath encompasses more than just the negative thoughts.

Find a situation that helps to support that. To do all that by yourself when you have cancer, of course, is asking a lot. It's possible, but it's asking a lot because usually, as human beings, we need some support. There are so many situations that call for this support. So to find a situation that's supported more than the old program - that maybe stops that from being possible. Sometimes, that means stepping away from the dynamics that we're caught up in - work, family, people, friends - and just taking a breather. They are caught up in the situation that's making everyone sick. So maybe if you get sick, you have to step aside and say, "Okay, now I need time for myself. I need the situation to support me." And not to have to put so much energy into all the other things that limit this oxygen from coming, this life force. Oxygen is life force coming into the physical organism, into supporting you.

Those steps are very hard to take because those steps usually mean that you have to look at so many other things. It's not as easy as saying, "Okay, I'll go on a holiday for a week." It requires a lot of changing, not just for you but also for all the people around you. But I think the people around, if they really love you - and really love you means showing it in a real sense - will support this in the end, because they will know that this is important. It's not just reacting from a negative, limited space, but also actually encompassing everything in a more positive way. A more positive way means everyone in the dynamics of what's going on opens up their hearts to support the person who has cancer. So the family gives more time to that person and gives more possibilities to that person. Work does the same. If people at work loved the person, they don't criticize or say, "This situation is so bad. I feel so sorry," but rather they do something that is positive to support the person to find a way to move himself out of that situation.

That is often what people fear when they have cancer. "What? I can't do this. It will hurt my partner. It will hurt my child. What will the people at work think? What will school think?" When they know that those people don't think anything negative or limiting, that they are part of the love and the communication, that allows a person to do their own thing. Then, I think there is a freedom that allows the cancer patient to breathe in more freely and then to breathe in more oxygen, more natural, vital energy.

For me, meditation is a fantastic thing, but only when put into practice. Again, there is time to consider. Time, when you have cancer, sometimes becomes more limited. So meditation in the East, as practiced in the East, requires a lot of time. People spend years doing this. So, I don't see it all the time as very relevant. So, in the courses that I do, for example, the meditations are totally changed to just sitting down and being quiet. This is ultimately the best. But by sitting down, it's not always easy to be quiet. What we're doing is not meditating, as such, in the sense of what's called deep meditation. We are just looking, gazing at our belly button or our navel. That sometimes is useful in the beginning, but I don't think it takes us to the point where meditation takes us. So, there are techniques of mediation that we can encompass in our daily life. That doesn't mean you have to go to a monastery or to Tibet or to Peru or wherever to sit down quietly and do whatever is necessary to meditate. For me, meditation is action. For example, it could be as simple as walking in the forest and just listening to the sounds, recognizing that there are more than the sounds of the mind. The birds sing. The wind blows through the trees. This helps us, the visualization of that, helps us to grow beyond the little circle that we could be caught up in - as we expand to love what is around us, love the beautiful sound of a bird or to be still enough to recognize nature. That expansion goes not only visually or in the senses, but also deep inside in our feelings and in the space that we create inside of ourselves. So that, of course, helps with the whole vital energy.

I suppose, if there is anything else to say, I would say a practical thing, another very important practical thing, is food, diet. I think it's a major aspect of healing. Whether you have a good diet or not such a good diet, it's important to look at how to utilize certain foods to help with the strengthening of the vital energy. Those vital foods are easy. They're foods that carry life energy. So basically, it's going back to a primitive diet and eating in a more healthy way.

It's amazing what eating healthy food can do to make you feel much better - inside physically but also on other levels, emotionally and energetically - which is important when you have cancer. That would be another practical thing that I would say is important for people to look at.

The last is love. It comes back down to the core of what it means to be alive and to find the love in every situation - not just in some situations, but every situation. I think the cancer can take you to certain situations that before were impossible to look at. When you can love the cancer for showing you that truth, then the love extends to those situations. Then you open your heart to such an extent that there will be no fear - if, for example, the cancer comes to a point where you die. There would be no fear in the situation of death because there will be so much love that carries you, transcends that limitation of the fear of death. That's important to know because I suppose this is in the back of people's mind - what happens if the cancer gets worse? I will die and what does that mean? Actually, you don't even have to think that because, if love fills the space, then there is no limited thoughts about what can happen - or what will happen or how am I going to react? There is just that moment of love. And people then recognize something that is so beautiful inside of you that love expands - to you and to all the people around.

http://www.tonysamara.org/

Made in the USA
Coppell, TX
16 March 2023

14306916R00105